BATTLING MELANOMA

BATTLING MELANOMA

One Couple's Struggle from Diagnosis to Cure

Claudia Cornwall

ROWMAN & LITTLEFIELD
Lanham • Boulder • New York • London

Published by Rowman & Littlefield
A wholly owned subsidiary of The Rowman & Littlefield Publishing Group,
Inc.
4501 Forbes Boulevard, Suite 200, Lanham, Maryland 20706
www.rowman.com

Unit A, Whitacre Mews, 26-34 Stannary Street, London SE11 4AB

British Library Cataloguing in Publication Information Available

Names: Cornwall, Claudia Maria, author.
Title: Battling melanoma : one couple's struggle from diagnosis to cure / Claudia Cornwall.
Description: Lanham : Rowman & Littlefield, [2016] | Includes bibliographical references and
    index.
Identifiers: LCCN 2016004054| ISBN 9781442245150 (cloth : alk. paper) | ISBN 9781442245167
    (electronic)
Subjects: : LCSH: Melanoma—Treatment. | Husband and wife.
Classification: : LCC RC280.M37 C67 2016 | DDC 616.99/477—dc23 LC record available at
    https://lccn.loc.gov/2016004054

∞ ™ The paper used in this publication meets the minimum requirements of
American National Standard for Information Sciences Permanence of Paper
for Printed Library Materials, ANSI/NISO Z39.48-1992.

Printed in the United States of America

We look for medicine to be an orderly field of knowledge and procedure. But it is not. It is an imperfect science, an enterprise of constantly changing knowledge, uncertain information, fallible individuals, and at the same time lives on the line. There is science in what we do, yes, but also habit, intuition, and sometimes plain old guessing. The gap between what we know and what we aim for persists. And this gap complicates everything we do. —Atul Gawande

CONTENTS

Acknowledgments   ix

Introduction: The Black Tumor   xi

1 A Pimple-like Thing   1

2 What's Real and What Isn't?   9

3 I Will Always Love You   25

4 The Mad Rush   31

5 Don't Worry About It   39

6 We Have No Way of Monitoring Success   53

7 The Iconoclast: A Visit with James Allison   65

8 A Cloud of Uncertainty   79

9 A Hairy Week So Far   87

10 It's Not Brain Surgery   99

11 The First Hill   107

12 Because I Am an Optimist   117

13 We Have Two Slots Left   133

14 An Unexpected Molecule   147

15 You've Got to Be Kidding!   159

16 Now, There Are All of You   175

Notes   189

Bibliography   203

Index   209
About the Author   213

ACKNOWLEDGMENTS

So many people helped to make this book possible. I'd like to thank my husband, Gordon Cornwall, for all he did to find a cure and to assist me in writing a book about it! I am indebted to Dr. Robert Scott, Dr. Youwen Zhou, Dr. George Chang, Dr. Charmaine Kim-Sing, Dr. Sasha Smiljanic, Dr. Ramesh Sahjpaul, Dr. Vivek Mehta, Dr. Sandra Vermeulen, Dr. Omid Hamid, and Dr. Anthony Tolcher for treating Gordon and talking to me about his case afterward. James Allison, Tasuku Honjo, Gordon Freeman, and Rafi Ahmed were generous with their time and gave me a better understanding of their research. Kathy Barnard, Shannon Gaudette, Yvonne and Bob Gerard, and Nigel Deacon provided a broader sense of the patient's point of view. Dr. Vanessa Bernstein added clarity about Nigel's struggles with melanoma. My daughter, Natalia Cornwall, and my son, Tom Cornwall, helped to keep me sane. My editor, Suzanne Staszak-Silva, showed extraordinary patience, and my agent, Robert Lecker, was encouraging.

INTRODUCTION
The Black Tumor

Melanoma. All those soft vowels and humming consonants make the word sound mellifluous—"dulcet, honeyed, soft, liquid, silvery, soothing, rich."[1] However, its meaning is anything but. The word comes from the Greek *melan,* for "black," and *oma,* for "tumor." Yes, *black tumor* is more like it. In European medical literature from the 1600s and 1700s, you can already find several references to "fatal black tumors with metastases and black fluid in the body."[2]

Melanoma is aggressive and can spread from the skin to almost any tissue, although the lungs, bones, abdomen, and brain are the likeliest targets. Until a few years ago, a diagnosis of metastatic melanoma was a death sentence. Physicians must have felt that we had made little progress since 1826 when Thomas Fawdington, an English doctor in Manchester, wrote:

> As to the remote and exciting causes of melanosis, we are quite in the dark, nor can more be said of the *methodus medendi.* We are hence forced to confess the incompetency of our knowledge of the disease under consideration, and to leave to future investigators the merit of revealing the laws which govern its origin and progress . . . and pointing out the means by which its ravages may be prevented or repressed. [3]

In 2012, when my husband, Gordon Cornwall, was told he had melanoma, I was both shocked and frightened. He was steadier than I was. "I'm healthy, strong. There is plenty of reason to hope," he said. And the situation—"the incompetency of our knowledge," as Fawdington described it—was beginning to change. Scientists were gaining a better understanding of the disease, of its defenses, and for the first time in history some people—a smattering of them—were surviving. But medicine was still in a state of flux. While life-saving treatments existed, accessing them was difficult. Gordon's oncologist could not simply write out a prescription for what he thought was best. We learned about "compassionate care," and about high-level negotiations between people we didn't know that might or might not grant Gordon an opportunity. So the prospect of a cure tantalized, but I was acutely aware that we might miss out. Sometimes I thought Gordon's life was hanging by a thread.

Melanoma is complicated, and Gordon saw several different physicians—his family doctor, dermatologist, surgeon, medical oncologist, radiation oncologist. We soon encountered an unexpected number of professional disagreements. I think this was partly because we were dealing with melanoma, which is, as I said, complicated, and partly because we were entering a new era, and the appropriate standard of care was not firmly established. Was a sentinel node biopsy a good idea? Would radiation boost long-term survival? When should systemic drug therapy be considered? What systemic treatment was available? Interferon? Or something more up to date? We heard different answers to all these questions. Gordon dubbed the proliferation of views "the fog of medicine." We relied on the intuitions of our family doctor, sought second and sometimes even third opinions. While we encountered disagreements that were unsettling, we also found wisdom and deep clinical experience that was invaluable. We did research on the web. In the process, we learned to appreciate the extent to which patients—with scientific papers just a few clicks away—can become partners in planning their own care. Realizing this is both empowering and overwhelming. You may suddenly find yourself saddled with more responsibility than you want.

We were in the middle of a medical paradigm shift. I sought to understand this, and was lucky enough to be able to speak to some of the scientists who made it happen. I learned that for the past hundred years, researchers had tried to enlist the immune system to eradicate cancers. After all, it destroyed pathogens such as viruses and bacteria. Melanoma, in particular, seemed a good candidate for this approach. Investigators had evidence that it was visible to the immune system and excited it—a first step. Moreover, they had nothing else. Chemotherapy had mostly dismal outcomes; melanoma could easily mutate its way out of that trap.

At first, researchers tried to "boost" the immune system in order to fight malignancies. This seemed like a good, commonsense idea, but these efforts did not work very well. A revved-up immune system can be quite toxic and only seems worthwhile for a few people. In general, the benefit is not worth the risk.

And then James Allison, a soft-spoken Texan, came along. He is a man who even as a teenager spoke his own mind. He did not suffer fools gladly—particularly fools in authority—and was always willing to go his own way, if he thought he was right. While others were trying to answer the question, "What turns the immune system on?" he became interested in a related but different inquiry, "What turns the immune system off?" This change in focus was surprisingly productive. Allison's answer to that question opened the door to a new drug. (Tasuku Honjo, a Japanese scientist, also answered the question and opened the door even further to additional therapies.) For his pioneering work, Allison is often called the father of immunotherapy. He has been honored with a blizzard of prestigious awards—to name a few, the Tang Prize for Bio-pharmaceutical Science, the Szent-Györgyi Prize for Progress in Cancer Research, the Canada Gairdner International Award, the Breakthrough Prize in Life Sciences, and the Lasker Award. Rumors abound that, one day, the Nobel may be his too.

Gordon and I have always been big boosters of our publically funded Canadian health care system. (For one thing, Americans spend about three times as much per capita on administration. We get more medicine for our buck.)[4] But any system has its downside, and one problem in Canada is long waiting lists. When you have cancer, waiting is hard; it is especially hard when your illness is melanoma, a malignancy that, given half a chance, will spread rapidly. On one occasion, desperate to know whether a certain lump was melanoma, we shelved our principles and traveled from our home in North Vancouver to Seattle. I phoned down on a Thursday, arranged for a scan the following Monday, and had results on the Tuesday—unfortunately yet again positive for melanoma. But in this way, we were able to speed up the removal of a tumor by several weeks.

In May 2013 the weather was glorious, but for us the days were dark. Gordon's scans kept getting worse and worse. *Game over*, I thought. But our oncologist, Dr. Sasha Smiljanic, encouraged us to keep fighting. We had run the gamut of approved treatments in Canada, so carrying on meant looking for a clinical trial. Gordon tried to enroll in a Canadian study several times but for various reasons was deemed ineligible. We began looking in the United States. I knew that because its population is ten times greater than our own, we were likely to find a better selection south of the border. But when we started the hunt, we had no idea whether Gordon would find that being Canadian was an impediment. Fortunately, it was not. Spots in trials were assigned to qualified patients on a first-come-first-served basis. The drug companies are interested in filling the studies without delay. From a research point of view, whether a patient is American or Canadian makes no difference. Still we felt we were being treated generously, and though it is painful for a good liberal Canadian to admit this, I must say that my feelings about Texas, where Gordon eventually found a clinical trial, have warmed up some!

The new knowledge we are acquiring about melanoma comes at a most opportune moment. According to the World Health Organization, it is one of the fastest growing cancers worldwide.[5] The incidence has increased by 253 percent among U.S. children and young adults since the 1970s, and young women appear to be especially vulnerable, accounting for two-thirds of cases diagnosed in 2011.[6] What lies behind these statistics is not entirely clear. Some researchers say they reflect better screening and earlier detection—that the number of people living with melanoma has not actually risen. Other investigators implicate the popularity of tanning beds or raise questions about the efficacy of sunscreens, which perhaps don't offer as much protection from harmful UV rays as they advertise. Obviously, more analysis is needed, but in the meantime, having better treatments can only be a good thing.

It is important to appreciate that immunotherapy doesn't succeed with everyone. As I write this, I am thinking about a young mother of three children under twelve. I met her just two weeks ago at a coffee party. She was receiving immunotherapy and radiation for her melanoma, and Dr. Smiljanic, who was also her oncologist, was optimistic. Although she seemed a little anxious, I thought she looked well. If you didn't know her history, you would not suspect that anything was wrong. The day after the party, she sent an e-mail to our hostess and the other guests, thanking them for "sharing their positive stories." And then last night, I heard that she had died—I can hardly believe it. We have more tools than ever to deal with melanoma, but it is still unpredictable and deadly. Physicians can't foresee who will profit from the new medicines. Searching for markers that will provide useful indications is an active area of inquiry. These signs will help them direct therapy where it will be most effective.

Gordon is now over two years past his last treatment. His scans have been good and we are cautiously optimistic. As I look back, I think that probably the most valuable lesson I learned was to search widely for resources to combat this deadly and difficult disease. According to Merriam-Webster, *crowdsourcing* (a business term coined in 2005) is defined as "the process of obtaining needed services, ideas, or content by soliciting contributions from a large group of people, and especially from an online community, rather than from traditional employees or suppliers."[7] We didn't use any crowdsourcing sites, but we made use of the technique nonetheless. We peppered our doctors with questions, and we found a group of knowledgeable melanoma survivors whose advice and support was invaluable. Their courage, often in the face of long odds, was inspiring. We traveled on a perilous journey, but in good company, and that made it better in so many ways.

I

A PIMPLE-LIKE THING

"It's not over," Gordon said as he walked in, his blue eyes serious, with no hint of a smile. His raincoat was spattered with drops of water, and mist clung to his curly hair. Behind him I could see our wooden porch, the boards glistening and wet. It was a drizzly, cold afternoon on March 1, 2012. Gordon closed the door behind him and gestured with a couple of sheets of paper. "Here's the pathology report." And then he paused before giving me the news. "It's melanoma."

"Melanoma!" I took a deep breath. The most serious kind of skin cancer. It could spread to many parts of the body and then you were in deep trouble. Did we catch it early enough? I had no way of knowing the answer to that question. I started to feel cold, and a tight knot formed in my stomach. Gordon put his arms around me and we stood together—silent for a moment, trying to collect ourselves. How strange it was, that everything could change so profoundly in just a day. Suddenly mortality was staring us in the face.

Beside us was a wall of family photographs—people and places—in no particular order. Our daughter, Talia, at age two, was smiling shyly, sitting on a log and wearing an outsize Greek fisherman's cap. We'd taken the kids canoeing in Johnstone Strait, off the northeast coast of Vancouver Island. While we were there, it rained every day, but we were rewarded by the sound of orcas breathing as they swam past our tent in the mornings. Talia's brother, Tom, about eight, was taking flight, laughing with delight as he jumped off a diving board into a pool near Vancouver's Jericho Beach, the blue North Shore Mountains in

the background. And there was Gordon, carrying a parachute and grinning, after his one and only sky dive. Horizon Aerosports 1982 Ltd. had
taken him following minimal training. Landing practice consisted of
leaping off a bench, and when Gordon hit the ground on the real dive,
he broke a bone in his foot—but was otherwise uninjured. I looked at
the pictures, as I did almost every day. *What's going to happen to us
now?*

"So the dermatologist was wrong," I said, easing myself out of Gordon's arms. "About the lump being squamous cell."

He shrugged, "People make mistakes."

I was less charitable. "How could you miss something like that?" And
then I asked, "What's next?"

"The surgeon says I need to come in again. Because he thought the
cancer was squamous cell, he took out a 1.2-centimeter margin of tissue
when he removed it. But for melanoma, the guidelines stipulate 2 centimeters. He has to take out more tissue."

"Did you tell him we were planning to go to Australia?"

Gordon nodded.

"Did he have a comment about that?"

"Not much of one. All he said was, 'Australia, huh?' And then he
indicated the surgery could wait. He booked the procedure for when
we get back."

We were due to leave our home in North Vancouver in three days
and stay away for nearly a month.

"Perhaps we should cancel our trip," I suggested.

"We don't have to do that," Gordon said. "Let's stick with the plan."
He was taking his cue from the surgeon, adopting the view that while
the findings weren't good, they weren't disturbing enough to make us
change course.

I thought, *This physician is so casual. His attitude seems inappropri-
ate, but what do I know? He's the expert, I'm just feeling my way.* I
didn't realize it then, but we had embarked on a journey that would
take nearly two years and for which no complete guidebooks were written. I would do a lot of feeling my way—trusting hunches, paying attention to a stirring in my stomach, catching a warning from telltales of
which I was not consciously aware.

The growth had appeared suddenly, three months before, in mid-December. In his diary, Gordon had written, *I noticed an elevated eruption on my left arm just above the elbow. I thought it was a pimple-like thing that would go away.* About the size of a small bean, it was quite hard, although it didn't hurt when Gordon touched it. Mostly he ignored it. Toward the end of December, at a blood donor clinic Gordon regularly attended, he got the first hint that something might be seriously amiss. When he proffered his arm, the nurse was obviously taken aback. "I'll have to ask my supervisor if you can still give blood," she said. After taking a quick look, the manager ruled that Gordon could donate, provided the needle went into his right arm. "But if it doesn't clear up soon" she advised, "you should see your doctor." That's when Gordon told me about it.

"You better go in right away," I said.

"Let's wait a bit," Gordon proposed. "Maybe it will resolve on its own."

A couple days later, a pleasant surprise: out of the blue, Zaya Benazzo, cofounder of SAND, the Science and Nonduality association, e-mailed Gordon from California. She told him she was organizing a conference called "The Nature of the Self." "Would you be interested in joining us and presenting your work?" Gordon had spent decades in the software industry, but in the summer of 2009, after selling his business, he decided to return to an old love of his—philosophy. He started a blog, *The Phantom Self*, to explore an idea he first encountered in a Buddhism class at the University of British Columbia (UBC) in1968.[1] He was tantalized by the possibility that many of the deep-seated beliefs we have about persons are illusions:

> Like the Phantom of the Opera, the self has a powerful voice that demands to be obeyed. Like an amputee's phantom limb, it is a vividly felt presence—but there is nothing really there.[2]

Zaya had never met Gordon, but she liked his blog and felt he could round out the speakers' roster. Gordon agreed to participate in the conference, which would be held in October, in San Rafael, just north of San Francisco. We decided it was a good excuse for a holiday in the Bay Area. I remembered earlier visits: shabby rooms with a grand view of the Golden Gate Bridge, a sultry Kurt Weill concert in a crowded nightclub, afternoons at Délices de France sampling buttery pastries.

Idly, I began to plan what we might see and do in the fall, and Gordon started writing an outline for his talk. However, the obdurate lump did go not away. In the middle of January, I remembered it with a start and prodded: "Gordon, how's that thing on your arm doing?"

He rolled up his sleeve. I glanced at the lesion, but what I saw so disturbed me, that I turned my head away abruptly. *It's growing and it's engorged with blood. That can't be a good sign.*

"It looks awful, Gordon."

"Okay, okay," he said. "I'll have it checked."[3]

Dr. Robert Scott has been a physician for thirty years and our GP for twenty of them. Slim with dark curly hair, he has a boyish appearance. But he cares deeply about the well-being of his patients. He hardly ever takes vacations, and his West Vancouver clinic is open seven days a week. Being a family doctor appealed to him, Rob once explained, "because it engages the whole spectrum of care. I couldn't imagine being an ear, nose, and throat specialist, or urologist, where you're just looking at one thing. It would be way too restrictive."

We like Rob even though he chides us about some of our choices—taking canoeing and kayaking holidays on the West Coast, for instance. He thinks this is dangerous—that we're tempting fate. But we love the freedom of it, wandering at will, camping on wild beaches, harvesting oysters, fishing for rock cod, swimming in the stunningly chilly water. There we live according to an older rhythm, governed by tides and the wind. I can never get enough of it. Gordon and I have both explained that we respect the weather; we recognize that our strength has limits. When it blows, we hole up, tuck ourselves safely away. Rob just shakes his head when we say this. We don't mind his caution though; we've agreed it's not a bad trait for your doctor to have.

Several times, I'd worried about small bumps on Gordon's skin and had asked him to show them to Rob. None proved to be a concern and he expected this one would be no different. But during all his years of medical practice, Rob had not seen anything like the angry pustule near Gordon's elbow. "Nasty," he concluded, and said, "It's likely a skin cancer." Then he referred Gordon to a dermatologist. "Probably a squamous cell carcinoma," she told Gordon. *So it's not nothing, after all,* he thought. When Gordon related the diagnosis to me, I was a little uneasy, but not overly alarmed. I knew we had to pay attention. But a squamous cell cancer wasn't likely to cause a problem. It was a minor nuisance, that's all. The dermatologist said it needed to be removed and that a plastic surgeon would do the excision.

A few days later, Gordon received a call: the procedure was scheduled for the beginning of March—two and a half months after he first noticed something. The lesion irritated him now, more psychologically than physically. Though he felt no pain, he was aware of the cancer and wanted to get rid of it, the sooner the better. Shortly after Gordon got the booking, he phoned back, "I was wondering," he said, "if you could put me on a wait list . . . in case there are cancellations." He was lucky. The local health authority had just granted the doctor an extra day for operations. That meant Gordon could come in two weeks earlier. "I'll be there," he promised.

As we were about to leave the house on the appointed day, Gordon said, "Wait a minute, I'd like to take a picture." I was startled. *Why does Gordon want to do that? The thing is so ugly . . . maybe if we needed a record . . . but that would mean . . .* I pushed the idea of future difficulties aside to some far corner of my mind. Watching Gordon getting out his camera reminded me that he is not nearly as squeamish as I am. He's the one who buries the rats that our cat, Charlie, kills on his night prowls and leaves as offerings in front of our bedroom door. In fact, Gordon has taken photos of some of these trophies. He likes to joke about submitting them for critique to his camera club along with the lovely shots of birds in flight at which many of the other members excel.

I drove Gordon to the hospital where he met the surgeon for the first time. He was rather brusque, and very efficient. In less than ten minutes, he was done and told Gordon to come back on March 1, to get the stitches out and review the biopsy. No big deal, his manner told us.

When Gordon arrived home on that dank March afternoon waving the report in his hand, I was completely unprepared for what it contained. I couldn't understand how Gordon could have melanoma. Sure he had moles, but this thing wasn't a mole and hadn't emerged from one. Gordon didn't seem to be particularly at risk for the disease either. He'd worked indoors most of his life. Nobody in his family had melanoma or any kind of cancer. In forty-one years of marriage, we'd only gone on one tropical vacation—to Maui with my parents. Gordon never tried purposefully to get a tan—and we lived on the slopes of Grouse Mountain, where it was even rainier than the rest of the Lower Mainland.

This new fact ripped through the fabric of my worldview, shredded it, leaving me feeling exposed and vulnerable. We didn't phone our kids right away—Tom, who was twenty-six, and Talia, who was twenty-four. We wanted to get used to what had happened first. We cooked dinner and shared a bottle of Gordon's blackberry wine. We'd picked the berries on the dike by the Fraser River near the airport, on a hot August day. Came home stained and scratched with a couple of buckets of the purple fruit. Gordon makes a dry rich wine—a distillation of coastal summer. He's made it since he was in his twenties, and long ago he designed a label for it and came up with a name—*In vino amor est:* "In wine there is love." After a few sips, I was calmer; even so, I kept running over the events of the last six weeks. Did I think that if I juggled them around enough, we'd get to a different result?

After supper, we cleaned up and went to bed. I don't know if it took me awhile to fall asleep, if I tossed and turned. But I do recall that in deepest night, around two or three, I woke suddenly, sat up in bed, and thought: *Gordon has melanoma.* The idea stained my consciousness, coloring everything. I was instantly wide awake and alert. My heart pounded. I had a sudden impulse to make sense of the pathology report. I didn't feel like waiting until morning. I wouldn't sleep anyway. I slipped out of bed quietly. The house was dark and cold as I padded down the hall to our office.

While my computer was booting up, I gazed at a small picture in a brown wooden frame: Gordon and I two years after we were married. In the summer of 1973, we were staying at his mom's cottage up north in the BC Cariboo. I was sitting on a diving board, legs outstretched, bare feet. Gordon was lying down on the board, his head in my lap. My arms were resting on his shoulders. I had chestnut hair then, long and curly. Gordon's hair was brown, long and curly too; he was bearded. He wore jeans with a red patch on one knee. I looked affectionately at the two young people. *We've loved each other for such a long time*, I reflected.

My desk was piled high with file folders stuffed with information for my current project. I felt weird as I looked at what I had been doing. A bit creepy. I wondered whether my work brought this on somehow.

And then I dismissed the notion. *That's crazy. It's just an uncanny coincidence.*

I was writing a book about cancers caused by infections. In fact, the impetus for our trip to Australia was to give me a chance to interview a couple of leading scientists in Perth. Only some cancers are caused by infections, and, as far as I knew, melanoma was not one of them. My manuscript had nothing to say about it and I had no special understanding of this malignancy. I was, however, used to reading medical reports and translating what I had learned into terms the general public could understand. So I was on familiar ground here. But on this occasion I had a personal stake in the results. So, was I hypersensitive to nuances in the data? Maybe. Did my emotional involvement cloud my judgment? Maybe that too.

I picked up the pathology report. Two pages, a small black typeface, an unprepossessing document for such momentous news. At the top it said, "Positive for invasive malignant melanoma, nodular type." *Invasive* and *malignant* were clearly worrying, but what was the significance of *nodular*? I consulted Google. I learned that while the majority of melanomas spread horizontally across the surface of the skin, a few grow vertically, often emerging where no previous lesion exists. They can penetrate the deeper layers of skin, invade the lymphatic system, and spread to other organs. Nodular melanomas account for about 15 percent of cases but nearly 40 percent of those that are fatal. Rapid growth is their hallmark. Unlike most melanomas, which are dark brown or black, they can be purple or pink. Their unusual appearance makes them hard to identify. Now I understood why even the dermatologist was fooled. And then I read about how long you had to react to this type of melanoma. I saw reports that some nodular melanomas "may take only six to eight weeks to develop significant life-threatening potential."[4] Of all the facts I uncovered, this one was the most devastating. Gordon's cancer had been removed just about eight weeks after he first noticed it. *So what does that do to his odds?*

Moving down to the next line of the report, I saw a number—"8.0 mm.," the "Breslow depth." I consulted various sources and learned that this was the height of the nodule from top to bottom. In 1970, Alexander Breslow, a pathologist at George Washington University, discovered the measurement was a reliable indicator of how well a patient would do. I came across tables illustrating that 95 percent of people with small melanomas, under a millimeter in depth, survived for five years after diagnosis. When their tumors extended farther, up to four millimeters, however, only 40 percent lived so long. I couldn't find specific data on eight-millimeter tumors, so I was left to speculate about the prognosis, but plainly "off-the-charts" couldn't be good. Finally, the pathologist had noted "ulceration." The skin on the surface was broken. It had a blistered, crusty appearance—evidence the malignancy was likely to spread. A bleak picture all-round.

The pathology report contained more information—something about the mitotic rate, a gauge of how fast the cells were dividing and growing, and something about staging of the melanoma. But I decided I had done enough research for one night. After over an hour of clicking away on the keyboard, sitting bathed in the computer's blue light, my heart stopped racing and the knot in my stomach dissolved. My body had prodded me into action and its work was done—I was taking the matter seriously.

The reconnaissance mission was worthwhile; I realized we were confronting a formidable force. Though shaken, I believed having a better sense of where we were would help us. I returned to our warm bed and fell asleep. When Gordon and I got up in the morning, I told him what I had discovered. "You know," I said, "nodular melanoma is very aggressive. It's the worst kind. I've bookmarked some sites if you want to see for yourself." And then for the second time, I proposed, "I think we should cancel that trip."

The lump had changed our lives utterly. But Gordon was unwilling to admit that. He paused before speaking. "Let's ask Dr. Scott," he suggested.

2

WHAT'S REAL AND WHAT ISN'T?

Gordon was reading on his iPad—a book by a Princeton philosophy professor, more research for his blog. I couldn't take in anything so challenging. Vainly, I tried to distract myself by leafing through a magazine, glancing at glossy pages displaying perfect kitchens. We were sitting in one of Dr. Scott's examination rooms, a drab cramped space with barely enough room for three people.

"What's going on?" Rob asked as he slipped into a chair. He opened his laptop and looked at Gordon expectantly.

"The skin cancer I saw you about . . . I'm supposed to have another excision, but we were planning to go away next week and I wondered . . ."

"Where were you thinking of going?" Rob asked.

"Australia," said Gordon.

"Australia?" Rob repeated.

Hearing the surprise in Rob's voice, Gordon felt he had to explain. "I'll be having the procedure when we get back in a month."

"I wouldn't go anywhere if I were you. I'd stay here and deal with this," Rob responded gravely.

Gordon caught my eye; we nodded to each other. It was pretty clear whose advice we were going to follow. Our intuitions lay with Rob. Later we would encounter other professional disagreements that were harder to sort out, but we didn't need to think this one over. Rob told us he'd like Gordon to see an oncologist—to explore further options. "What about someone in the Melanoma Clinic at the BC Cancer Agency?" I asked. "That's a good idea," he said. After promising we'd get an appointment in a few days, he patted Gordon on the back and was gone, on to the next patient.

We were quiet for a few minutes, adrift in our own thoughts. Then as Gordon began driving home, he said, "Even if I stay, you can still go. You could do your interviews."

"And leave you, at a time like this?"

"It's only a few days. I'll be all right,"

"But I wouldn't be. I'm not going anywhere."

How fortuitous it was, I thought, that Gordon had pushed his surgery ahead. If he hadn't, we'd have no biopsy results now. We'd be en route to Australia in two days, about to drink in all that southern sunshine, probably not a good idea, considering. And Gordon's second surgery wouldn't happen until April, probably not wise either.

We unraveled our travel plans, canceled our flights and hotels. I sent an e-mail: "My husband has had a sudden and serious health issue. . . ." I told Gordon I was considering giving up my book. He protested forcefully, "I don't want you hovering over me!" I replied equally vigorously, "I'm not hovering!"

And then I phoned our kids: "We're not going to Australia, after all. . . ." In the evening, they came over to spend some of the weekend with us. Tom, who is married, was studying economics at UBC, and Talia was working for Raincoast, a local book distributor. I felt fortunate that they weren't at the other end of the country. We played bridge—a favorite activity of ours on kayaking trips. During heavy weather, we've whiled away many an hour playing cards. Old habits are soothing, but the problem that drew us together had not gone away.

At one point when I was alone with Tom, he told me with tears in his eyes, "It's hard to say this, but I don't think Dad has much time left." I could see that he, too, had been googling. Then he went on, "I hope he doesn't have to spend all of that time in doctors' offices and appointments—that he gets to go to California."

"I hope so too," I said. I knew the conference in San Rafael meant a lot to Gordon. His ideas on the nature of the self are unorthodox, and he was excited about the opportunity to communicate them and meet like-minded people. I asked Tom, "How much time do you think he has, a year?"

Tom said, "That's what I've been thinking."

On Saturday evening, we all went to a contest hosted by Gordon's camera club. Gordon's entry showed our cat, Charlie, greatly blown-up in size, stalking two tiny people walking along the Stanley Park Seawall. Gordon's fondness for "altered reality" made him something of an odd man out in the competition; most of the other participants were accomplished nature photographers. Nevertheless, Gordon won the People's Choice Award, which buoyed our spirits considerably. Sunday morning, he cooked waffles—a weekend tradition he inherited from his mother. Life did not seem quite so dire as we handed around bowls of fruit, maple syrup, and a large pot of coffee. After Tom and Talia left, Gordon wrote in his diary:

> *March 4. The kids came clustering around on Friday and stayed yesterday, and we're having dinner together again tonight. Their love for me shines through. Claudia frets too much, of course. I am blessed in my family!*

I too took up my pen, but less cheerfully:

> *March 4. I am a wreck. Couldn't sleep much last night. My life is unravelling. Gordon is remarkably steadfast. I say, "I'm afraid." He says, "You're afraid I will die. But I don't think so. I'm healthy, strong. There is plenty of reason to hope." But melanoma is tough. Very little chemotherapy seems to work.*

I had become obsessed with the idea that we had lost valuable time. So first thing on Monday, I called the surgeon's office. I asked about getting an earlier date for Gordon's excision—since we weren't going on our trip, after all.

"Actually," the receptionist said, "there's a spot later this week, on Wednesday."

"We'll take it!" I exclaimed, and so succeeded in getting the procedure bumped ahead by four weeks. Our decision to give up on the trip was already bearing fruit. I felt better—because I could act. But the next day, I was worrying again:

> *March 6. Gordon tells me not to expect the worst. Unfortunately, that's what I do. I berate myself for not looking at the Internet earlier! I feel we were too late. Too much noodling around because of the*

wrong squamous cell diagnosis. Obituaries are running through my head. It's awful. Gordon says it's too soon to gather round his bed with lilies! We share a laugh now and again.

"This melanoma," Gordon said while the surgeon was setting up for the second excision in the outpatient clinic, "was pretty high risk—eight millimeters deep and ulcerated." Vivid in Gordon's mind was an experience a friend of ours went through a couple years before. She had breast cancer, and the surgeon who was supposed to remove it operated on the wrong breast. Three weeks later, the surgeon tried again; she got the right breast but didn't manage to take out the malignant tissue. She only succeeded on the third attempt. Gordon hoped to avoid such distress.

"It was *zero point eight*," the doctor stated emphatically.

"*Eight point zero* millimeters." Gordon insisted.

The surgeon made a phone call to check. "He was out by an order of magnitude," Gordon reported, when he told me the story afterward. Perhaps that's why he seemed so nonchalant about the idea of us taking off for a month. In any case, his misapprehension strengthened our inclination to take an active role in what was going on.

A couple of nights later, as we lay under a reproduction of Gustav Klimpt's painting "The Kiss"—a man and a woman embracing, swathed in gold—hanging on our wall, I was conjuring up specters. Gordon was asleep, but I was thinking about our visit to the BC Cancer Agency the following afternoon. I had a sinking feeling about it. I flinched from the prospect. I expected being there would make me depressed. What could we learn? More devastating statistics? The word *riddled* came up, and I visualized being told the cancer had spread throughout Gordon's whole body. There was no evidence of this, but I concocted the scenario and became anxious anyway. Then I remembered how I had always been frightened of rounding Rafael Point on Flores Island when we kayaked in Clayoquot Sound. We'd get to Cow Bay and I wouldn't want to go any farther north. I used to refer to "dreaded Rafael Point" because our guidebook warned that paddling past it "can be harrowing" and intoned, "There are no safe landings between the point and Siwash Cove. You are 100 percent committed out there and will feel it."[1] I always pictured us beating our way around in the teeth of the wind. But one day, I agreed to give it a go. As we reached the point that had figured so intensely in my imagination, the sea was flat and grey— benign. I reflected that things do not always turn out as badly as I imagine. My fears ebbed away.

Dr. Youwen Zhou, a dermatologist who also had a PhD in molecular genetics, took our appointment at the BC Cancer Agency. At first, I was disappointed Gordon wasn't seeing an oncologist. I thought Rob had intended he should. Then I decided that if the BC Cancer Agency had selected Dr. Zhou, he was probably the right person for us to consult. I had formed a favorable impression of the agency while working as a freelance writer on health issues. British Columbia enjoyed the lowest death rates from cancer in Canada, and I was convinced the work the agency did to prevent and treat malignancies was a contributing factor. In BC, breast cancer mortality began to decline a decade earlier than elsewhere in the world. By the 1990s physicians were aware that adding chemo and hormone therapy to surgery could save lives. The discovery made more of an impact in BC than in other places, however, because the BC Cancer Agency centralized its policies so that patients all over the province would have the same innovative treatments.[2] I told myself we were in good hands and that I should relax. However, while walking through the heavy steel door between the parking garage and the agency, I was on edge. I felt I had crossed a divide into an alien and forbidding territory.

After Gordon reported to the front desk, he sat down and filled out a few forms concerning his health history, including one about his stress levels. As he worked through the questions, I read some of them: "Are you jittery?" "Is it hard for you to concentrate?" "Are you bothered by black thoughts?" Gordon dutifully ticked off boxes labeled from 1 to 5 to indicate how much of a problem he was having. He chose box 1 (least stress) for most of them. I laughed and told him that I would have checked off 5 to nearly every one.

A few minutes later, we entered a cell-like room, no window, no pictures on the walls, nothing to draw me away from those black thoughts to which that questionnaire referred. "Did you bring something to read?" Gordon asked. I shook my head. I was too nervous to read. Then Dr. Zhou stepped into the room, smiled broadly, introduced himself, and shook our hands. A man in his forties, he seemed serene and self-confident. He wanted to know what brought us to see him and so Gordon pulled out the photograph of his arm and began telling his story. When he finished his account, Dr. Zhou glanced at Gordon's yellow file folder, thick with papers, studies, options. "You've been doing your research?" We both nodded. "Good," he said. "Do you have some questions for me?" Of course we did.

"Do you think I should have a sentinel node biopsy?" Gordon asked. A sentinel node is the first lymph node to receive lymph fluid in the area around a tumor. If it is infected, this could mean the cancer will spread and that surgery to remove more lymph nodes may be in order. The technique has been used fairly routinely in the treatment of melanoma since the early 1990s. But Dr. Zhou said, "I don't recommend it."

"Why is that?" I inquired.

"We do it for patients with smaller tumors. But when people have large ones, the biopsy doesn't give us additional information or increase patients' chances of long-term survival," he explained. I was surprised, but I accepted what Dr. Zhou said. I understood that you had to weigh the evidence. You had to follow its lead.

"Well then, what about drug treatments?" Gordon asked.

Dr. Zhou shook his head. "I wouldn't advise them unless there's clinical evidence of disease elsewhere in your body that can't be treated with surgery. Now you need close monitoring, that's all." Gordon and I did not question Dr. Zhou's advice; we were thankful that Gordon could avoid a disagreeable therapy.

"Some of my patients have lived for decades after a diagnosis like yours—without any further treatment," Dr. Zhou added.

I took a deep breath. A few of the dark clouds hanging over our heads since my late-night study of the pathology report were dispersing. Then, Dr. Zhou gave Gordon a skin examination. More good indicators: he had no other suspicious lesions, in general little skin damage, and normal lymph nodes.

"Is there anything else?" Dr. Zhou asked.

Gordon did have one last question: "The pathology report indicated I was stage four. I wondered what my prognosis is?"

Dr. Zhou looked puzzled for a minute and then said, "Your *tumor* is stage four, but *you* are stage two because, as far as we know, the melanoma has not spread." In other words, Gordon's condition was markedly less perilous than we thought. We hadn't understood the rather complicated system used to classify melanoma. Later we read that tumors are assigned numbers from one to four (often written as Arabic numerals) based on their size and other characteristics. Patients are also assigned numbers from one to four (usually written as Roman numerals). If their lymph nodes are involved, they are stage III, and if the disease has infected other organs, they are stage IV. Gordon's melanoma was large, so that put him in stage II, but no higher, because he had only one tumor, and his lymph nodes were not affected. He was a whole two stages less advanced than we had previously thought—a marked improvement.

Dr. Zhou wanted Gordon to have a chest X-ray and some blood tests before he left the agency. He said that Gordon should come back in three months, but if we had any concerns before that appointment, we should phone his office. "I'll return your call right away," he pledged.

We left feeling considerably more upbeat than when we had arrived. Dr. Zhou's suggestion that no further action was necessary put my mind at rest. In fact, my mood had improved so much I thought a minor celebration was in order. I invited my mother to join us for lunch at her favorite restaurant, a tiny tea shop, not far from her house. We had the usual lox and cream cheese on focaccia bread, followed by Darjeeling tea.

Two years later, when I talked to Dr. Zhou about this early appointment, he added to my understanding of sentinel node biopsies. Again, he said they were considered helpful for smaller tumors. Positive results would indicate a higher level of risk and negative ones, a lower level. The tests provided more information. But large tumors like Gordon's were dangerous, regardless of the outcome of a sentinel node biopsy. A negative test wouldn't change the assessment significantly. Nothing was gained by performing the biopsy. I must admit that during our visit with Dr. Zhou, I didn't grasp Gordon's circumstances correctly. I took them to be more encouraging than they really were.

In any case, back in March 2012, the day after we saw Dr. Zhou, my optimism evaporated. I started to wonder whether I was experiencing more reassurance than was warranted. I had been scouring the Internet for resources and found the Melanoma Network of Canada, a patient advocacy group based in Toronto. I e-mailed Annette Cyr, a melanoma survivor and founder of the network. She replied right away. "I would definitely ask why there is no sentinel node biopsy. I would also wonder why a CT scan and MRI wasn't done. Usually a CT scan would be ordered, not just chest X-ray. If there is no further spread into the lymph nodes, the standard of care is 4 weeks of high dose interferon followed by another 11 months of low dose self-injections. Only if a patient is elderly or has other health issues would they likely not mention it." Annette's note left me with more questions than answers. The "wait and see" approach advocated by Dr. Zhou had made me happy, sounded like good news. But I began to worry that we were not doing enough.

Gordon went to see Rob again to discuss his options. He explained that he liked Dr. Zhou and felt awkward asking for a second opinion about the sentinel node biopsy and possible drug treatments. But still he wondered whether it might be worthwhile. "Don't feel awkward," Rob said. "It's your life." Rob told Gordon he would refer him to Dr. Sasha Smiljanic, an oncologist who practiced in North Vancouver. Gordon had one more question. He had been reading a book called *Beating Melanoma* by an oncologist at the Sloan Kettering Cancer Center in New York. In it, the author, Steven Wang, referred to a study indicating that about a quarter of melanoma pathology reports were incorrect. Errors crept in, particularly if general pathologists did the work, rather than dermatopathologists (who specialize in skin disorders).[3] "Should we have the results reviewed?" Gordon asked. "You can put in a request to the BC Cancer Agency," Rob remarked, "but I don't think they'll agree." Despite Rob's reservations, Gordon phoned Dr. Zhou, to gauge his views about that second appraisal. Dr. Zhou liked the idea and said he'd order it.

The lack of consensus was unsettling, because the choices mattered. Make the wrong one and the melanoma might get the upper hand. Somehow Gordon and I would have to navigate through the confusion. But how? From an early age, I had learned that information was your friend. I remembered an argument I had with my father about marijuana. He mentioned newspaper stories about the dismal effects of smoking it. I took the position that the articles were overblown. We were at an impasse. The discussion was obviously leading nowhere, so my dad said, "I'm going to the library." Not one to procrastinate, he left right away and a couple of hours later returned with an armful of books. I actually don't recall what was in those books or whether they helped to resolve our disagreement. But my father's strategy made a big impression on me: cast your net wider. So that's what I did. I looked for more data. I discovered another organization dedicated to supporting patients and educating the public about skin cancer. This one, called Save Your Skin, was conveniently located in North Vancouver, where we lived. I e-mailed the founder, Kathy Barnard, also a melanoma survivor, to find out more about how she managed to defeat the disease. She replied immediately: "Please call me."

A few days later, Gordon and I met Kathy in a local café. An athletic-looking woman with shoulder-length blond hair, she smiled readily and spoke with rapid-fire eagerness to impart what she knew. As we sat on rickety stools around a small round table listening to Kathy talking about her experiences, I was completely engrossed. The busy coffee shop clatter faded, and it was as if there were only the three of us in the room. "They gave me six months to live," she said.

Kathy's story began more than a decade ago, in 2002, when she noticed a lump near her elbow. "My family physician thought it was just fatty tissue, nothing significant." Kathy kept asking about the growth, until finally the doctor sent her to a plastic surgeon. On Mother's Day, 2003, Kathy got the news: she had malignant melanoma. Immediately, she was referred to Dr. Paul Klimo, a North Vancouver oncologist. He ordered radiation and a course of interferon, an early immunotherapy. Interferon is a protein the body makes in small amounts to fight infections and tumors. Researchers had turned it into a medicine by cloning it and giving patients amplified amounts; they thought this might boost the body's native cancer-fighting capacity. Interferon helped Kathy for a while, but in March 2005 she developed a fourteen-centimeter mass in one lung. Dr. Klimo ordered chemotherapy, but Kathy did not respond to it. She decided to consult another doctor for a second opinion. He gave her his heart-wrenching opinion: she didn't have long to live. At that point, Kathy's son, who didn't accept this verdict, found a newer immunotherapy called interleukin-2. It was available on an experimental basis from an American doctor who was willing to send it to Canada. Dr. Klimo was in favor of trying the medicine, but he did not have a facility where interleukin-2 could be administered safely. He arranged for Kathy to see Dr. Michael Smylie, an oncologist at the Cross Cancer

Institute in Edmonton and western Canada's foremost expert on melanoma. Dr. Smylie was able to give Kathy the infusion. Interleukin-2 is similar to a protein that we all produce naturally when struggling with disease. However, in the amounts deemed necessary for a successful therapy it can have devastating side-effects. Kathy almost died from it. "I code blued," she said.

The medication controlled the melanoma for about a year, but in 2007 it came back as a nine-centimeter mass in Kathy's bowel. After the tumor was removed surgically, Dr. Smylie suggested Kathy have an even newer immunotherapy, which we now call ipilimumab (or Yervoy), to make sure the cancer didn't return. It was less toxic than either interferon or interleukin-2 and also more effective. Although not approved for general use in Canada at the time, the developer, Bristol-Myers Squibb (BMS), was letting Dr. Smylie give it to a few patients. Kathy credits ipilimumab with saving her life. She was one of the first Canadians to survive metastatic melanoma. "I'm beginning to think I may be cured," she said, grinning widely.

I liked Kathy's attitude. Matter-of-fact and direct, she seemed to take the view that a diagnosis of melanoma was serious, but she didn't invest the disease with a kind of demonic power, which is what I tended to do. Her manner and her tone of voice signified we had cause for concern, but no reason to be terrified. I learned several important lessons from Kathy. I came to understand that fighting melanoma could be a long campaign, but even if you lost a skirmish or two you could still win the war. I saw that the world of melanoma was changing rapidly, but to take advantage of medical breakthroughs, we might have to travel. I also concluded that we would probably have to find those possibilities ourselves and not rely on our doctors to do the legwork for us.

Kathy was proactive and encouraged us to be so as well. She suggested Gordon ask to have his tumor tested to see whether it was positive for a BRAF mutation, a faulty gene that contributed to rampant cell growth.[4] Zelboraf, a new drug recently approved by Health Canada, shrank tumors by interfering with this gene. "Just in case," she said. "If the melanoma doesn't come back, you won't need this information. But if does, you'll be ready." She explained that if the tumor was BRAF negative, it might still be positive for another growth-stimulating gene called C-KIT. If so, other drugs might help. And then she gave us her last and best news: Health Canada had approved ipilimumab the previous month. The BC Cancer Agency was still doing its due diligence to determine whether it would pay for the treatment. But in the meantime, Kathy assured us, there was a good chance BMS would provide the drug through its compassionate care program—until the BC Cancer Agency made its final decision.

Melanoma was as deadly as ever. But we had many more tools at our disposal than Kathy had when she was first diagnosed. She made me feel quite hopeful. We left after telling Kathy we would keep her posted on Gordon's progress. I felt we had an important ally. I wrote earlier that we had no guidebooks for the voyage we were on, and that was still true, but I was discovering that we could rely on pilots who knew the local waters. In the months that followed we would turn to Kathy again and again for her advice and the benefit of her experience.

I was staring out the window as Gordon told his story to an oncologist. Dr. Smiljanic, to whom he was originally referred, was away for a few weeks, so he was seeing someone else. Gordon pulled out his shot of the melanoma and pushed it across the desk. As those two bent over the color print, I found refuge in the sky: I stared out the window. I hated looking at the dark-red pustule. It always distressed me. I thought of the nodule as my mute and deadly enemy.

Gordon opened the binder he had started recently—*The Melanoma Record*. It contained a list of appointments and procedures, and what had transpired at each one. He also included copies of reports and biopsies and the like. Gordon had always used binders to organize his working life. At his company, Industrial Metrics, he had binders for accounting, binders for projects, binders for research, binders for customers. Binders came naturally to him.

Referring to this log, Gordon spoke about his two excisions, his meeting with Dr. Zhou, and our burgeoning list of questions. The oncologist listened carefully and said, "You know if I were in your shoes, I'd want a sentinel node biopsy—even if it doesn't have a survival benefit. I'd do it for planning purposes." *That was an interesting point,* I thought. Survival wasn't the only consideration. Making the most of the life one had left was also important.

Gordon agreed. He said, "I'd like that."

"I'll refer you to a local surgeon."

Then Gordon asked, "What about drug therapy?"

"Let's wait for the result of the sentinel node biopsy." The specialist advised, "If it is positive," she said, "we can talk about interferon."

This was the drug Kathy had back in 2004. I had been reading about it recently and learned that while early studies looked promising, later research showed patients who got it did not do much better than patients who received nothing. After our conversation with Kathy, I had come to assume that we were now into an era of new drugs for melanoma. "What about ipilimumab?" I asked. The doctor repeated what I already knew—that despite Health Canada's endorsement, the BC Cancer Agency had not yet decided to fund it. "At the moment," she said, "interferon is pretty much it." *But Kathy received ipilimumab years ago,* I thought to myself. I was convinced that something else besides interferon was available. I didn't know how we would get it, but I was determined to try.

That evening, I was anxious. Dark fears scudded through my mind; I had trouble sleeping. Next morning, after breakfast, I felt Gordon was upset and asked, "Is something wrong?" We are pretty sensitive to each other's moods. In fact, we often made fun of this. I would say, "You're happy today," and Gordon would respond, "Good to know, good to know."

We were standing in the middle of our office, our two desks on one side, a wall of books on the other. Gordon looked at me intently. "Last night," he said, "while we were in bed, I noticed this lump, under the skin." He rolled up his sleeve and pointed. I could see that it wasn't far away from the site of the original melanoma.

"Oh no," I said. *This is game over,* I thought, considering the implications of another growth emerging just six weeks after the first one was removed. The by-now-familiar battery of reactions fired up: racing heart, knotted stomach, a shivery cold feeling. So odd, I thought, that I had been fearful last night. I wondered whether I had already been aware of something wrong. I wouldn't have been able to articulate anything. But did I have a perception of some sort? Obviously, it was important to remain alert, pay attention to just such inchoate warnings.

"It could be a cyst," Gordon said.

"I don't know. That seems unlikely under the circumstances. I think you need a biopsy."

"Yeah, I'll call."

I didn't have to press. Even Gordon was shaken by the development. He wrote:

March 28. Nothing like the diagnosis of a life threatening disease to make self-concern kick in. I can use this as refresher course in the phenomenology of the self-directed emotions—the somatic symptoms, the anxious virtual pacing back and forth between the walls of thought. Last night in bed I found a hard little lump on my arm, below the skin, seemingly attached to the muscle. In the shower this morning I couldn't find it. Such an event wouldn't have worried me at all before this melanoma scare. The threat is not clear and obvious, like an aggressive person, or a stiff wind when you're on the water— it lies within your body, mostly hidden, and makes wonderful fodder for the imagination.

My blog numbers are down lately. I haven't been getting as much done—although I've made a good start on my talk for San Rafael! Pulled this way and that—that is the human condition. I believe I have a contribution to make, but I frequently feel that no one will ever get it. The human mind is designed (by natural selection) not to get it.

And yet, to a large extent, I get it and so I persevere. Understanding the self allows me to manage it rather than being managed by it. (Can that paradox be sorted out?)

I was, as usual, focused on the present danger:

March 29. I have to face this. Be clear-eyed and strong. Don't cringe. Above all, don't cringe.

I told Gordon I was giving myself pep talks and he responded by trying to give me one himself.

"If I die," he said, "you'll be okay, you have the kids."

"It's not the same," I said.

"I know, but on the scale of human tragedies, it would have been worse if this had happened fifteen years ago."

Nothing. Gordon left another message for the oncologist.

Still nothing.

"Why don't you call Dr. Zhou," I suggested. Gordon did that, and on April 2, Dr. Zhou phoned back. He told Gordon to see him for a biopsy of the new lump. He also said the pathology review had confirmed the original diagnosis of melanoma. *Damn*, I thought.

> *April 3. Gloomy phrases pounding through my brain. Don't like to write them down—makes them more real. Afraid this will make them come true. Ridiculous thinking. If it were that easy to influence reality, one could do the reverse, write down a lot of positive outcomes, and bring that about.*

> *April 4. Gordon somewhat low-spirited. I think he's finally seeing the stats might apply to him. But he still thinks his chances might be better than others because of his age, life style, and general good health. I tell him that we will be very lucky if the melanoma hasn't spread. He says that is my doom voice talking. Dunno. What's real and what isn't?*

When we saw Dr. Zhou on the afternoon of April 4, he told us Gordon had two options: a needle biopsy, in which a few cells are extracted, or a surgical removal of the whole lump. The latter procedure was preferable because the test (of a larger amount of tissue) was more reliable. Since the growth was close to the surface of Gordon's arm, excision was possible, and Dr. Zhou decided to do it right then and there. I was delighted Gordon would be leaving the office lump-free. Had the lesion been deeper inside his body, Dr. Zhou would have had to perform a needle biopsy. That route to treatment was glacially slow. We'd have to wait for the pathology report and then, if positive, wait again for a surgery date. The process could easily take three to four weeks, a delay we preferred to avoid. After Dr. Zhou completed the excision, he said, "It's a swollen lymph node. It could be reacting to disturbance in the area—to the surgery, the removal of stitches—or it could be infected with melanoma. The odds are about fifty-fifty."

I didn't like those odds much. But I was grateful to Dr. Zhou for his speedy response. It was interesting, I reflected. When we were in a quandary about the sentinel node biopsy, we had turned to the oncologist and found her advice sensible. But she had disappointed us by being unavailable in response to this new threat. There Dr. Zhou shone. It seemed that no one person had a monopoly on the truth or the best course of action. While we were waiting for the next pathology report, we finally heard from the cancer specialist. She apologized for not getting in touch sooner: somehow Gordon's messages got lost in her system. Gordon told her the growth he had described in his message was out and that he was waiting for the result of the biopsy. I wrote:

> *April 6. I have a kind of short-hand now. Instead of saying, "I don't like going through this," I say "A." Instead of "I'm so worried or so afraid," I say, "B." It makes us both laugh a little. I forget what "C" is. A & B pretty well cover it. A! B!*

And Gordon wrote:

> *April 7. I feel in limbo, and angry about it. I don't know how to plan my life. Should I go all out on the book? Sometimes that feels right.*

In the fall of 2011, Gordon had started writing a book based on his blog, but he still had much to do on it. Now, with the future so up in the air, he was in a dilemma. Did such an undertaking make sense anymore?

The report we wanted came on April 13—Friday the 13th. Dr. Zhou told us the new lump was positive for melanoma. Because of that, he was ordering a PET scan to see whether the disease had spread any further. I wrote:

> *I had a doomy feeling about that lump. Gordon says, "You and your doomy feelings." He smiles, looks cheerful. I'm glad it was removed so quickly. But SHIT! If only Gordon had gone to the doctor earlier in the first place. We might be further ahead. "We look before and after/ And pine for what is not." I asked Gordon if he considered there was a chance the PET scan would be negative. He thought there was. He said in fact, that he expected it. True to form, I was less optimistic. I felt all my earlier fears and forebodings were borne out. I was afraid of a long lonely future. How can I live without Gordon? I hear him saying, "I'm still here!" That's important to remember. But how much time do we have left?*

3

I WILL ALWAYS LOVE YOU

The trip to Seattle was our daughter-in-law's idea. A girls' weekend away. Leanna invited Talia, a couple of friends, and me. I said I'd enjoy coming, but I wasn't going to leave Gordon behind—not when things were so uncertain. So he joined us, in an honorary capacity. On Saturday, we wandered—past the Experience Music Project, a pop culture museum that had rippling lines evoking a smashed guitar. Then we explored the Pike Street Market with its towering displays of fresh fish—scampi, lobster tails, scallops, king crab and Dungeness, Copper River salmon, tuna, cod, snapper, sole. We walked uptown to the Byrnie Utz hat store, a Seattle institution founded in 1934, where I hoped to find an Indiana Jones–style fedora for Gordon. Since he now had to wear a hat when he went outdoors, I thought he might as well look good in it. The shop had a wide selection—Stetsons, bowlers, berets, boonies, top hats, trilbys, porkpies, homburgs, Panamas, even boaters—and we soon found what we were looking for, in chocolate brown felt. On Sunday, we browsed at the Elliott Bay Book Company, an independent bookstore where you can lose yourself for hours. We carried on to the Central Library, an architectural landmark, designed by Rem Koolhaas. We gazed up at its grand atrium, inspected a four-story spiral containing the nonfiction book collection, rode the chartreuse escalator, and strolled along blood-red corridors shaped like intestines. And then on a walkway near the roof of the atrium, I took a picture of Gordon in his new hat.

For the whole weekend, Gordon and I hardly thought about melanoma. We didn't talk about lumps or bumps or doctors or scans or what his outlook was. We acted like normal people whose most serious problem concerned which restaurant to pick for dinner. But once home, we went back at it. Gordon saw Dr. George Chang, a surgeon, to discuss a possible sentinel node biopsy. Three weeks ago, this had seemed like a good idea to us, but since then the disease had progressed. Dr. Chang decided the biopsy was no longer necessary. In effect, Dr. Zhou had already performed the procedure when he removed the infected lymph node from Gordon's arm. That told us what we needed to know—the melanoma was spreading. Gordon's upcoming PET scan would tell us more.

April 18. Yesterday I felt weirdly okay—not nervous. I kept saying to Gordon, "I'm not worrying. I should be worrying. If I don't worry, I'll pay for it later. I have to suffer." This is irrational. My state of mind has nothing to do with what's going on inside Gordon's body. But there it is. Today the familiar symptoms—faster heartbeat, butterflies in the stomach. I'm a bit shaky. At least, I don't have to worry that I'm not worrying enough!

I had always believed Gordon and I were likely to live together many years. We were close in age (I was younger by just nine months), and until recently, both of us felt healthy. But the road to the future on which we were both walking seemed to be getting shorter. I was drawn to thinking about the past—our happy shared past.

I went to the same high school as Gordon did, and he always says he first noticed me in grade 9 because of a crocheted sweater that my grandmother had made for me. It had a way of slipping off my shoulder that he liked. We didn't speak to each other much at first, but we became friends in grade 12. We were part of a philosophy club that met about once a week. Five or six of us stayed after school, looked for a quiet room somewhere, and had a discussion. One afternoon, the vice principal discovered our meeting and told us we were doing something highly irregular. Our so-called club had no sponsoring teacher and therefore we had no right to be in the building. We had to get out. Well, we didn't get out. We found another room—the teachers' lunchroom, of all places, and carried on. For some reason, lost in the mists of time,

Gordon was lying on a table declaiming about an idea that interested him. It might have been the notion that gripped his imagination then that human beings are essentially selfish, even when they perform acts of kindness. I can't be sure that was his subject, although I do know that the vice principal, upon hearing the clamor, came over to investigate. This was our second transgression, and therefore more serious. But we were in the dying days of our grade 12 year and perhaps the vice principal didn't see the point of a big confrontation. In any case, he let us off with a warning, saying if we didn't get out immediately, he would have to punish us. Reluctantly, we left. I remember muttering about the irony of being kicked out of school when we were trying to learn.

Gordon and I stayed friends and kept talking. We both entered the Faculty of Arts at the University of British Columbia (UBC). Our first fall there, it rained for forty days straight—or maybe almost forty days. I had two pairs of boots; I would wear one pair and then the other, but they never dried out. So I have a memory of wet feet, and awful coffee and long conversations. We used to rail about the evils of materialism while having lunch together; we still do this occasionally and laugh. Some things never change.

I was seeing our life as a kind of tapestry—the good and the bad woven together, light strands richly illuminating the dark. "Dear Gordon," I wrote on the afternoon of April 19, starting what turned out to be quite a long letter:

> I do not understand your equanimity at all! I do remember the times when you were worried about your business affairs, and I cannot comprehend why you were more anxious then than now. It seems to me that much more is at stake now! What, after all, is a business in trouble in comparison with this?
>
> You say that if you had faced a melanoma diagnosis ten or fifteen years ago, it would have been much more difficult for me. It is true. I would have had much more to cope with financially. And parenting is so much easier and more agreeable when there are two of you to take a hand at it.
>
> But still! I look forward at the prospect of life without you and it seems bleak indeed. Empty—without your love, your counsel, your support. I think of all the things we have done together. That magical trip up Sechelt Inlet, one of our very early ones, where we camped on the thick moss on the point, and swam at night, naked in the

phosphorescent water. I felt like Tinker Bell, as I thrust out my arms and thousands of stars flew out from my fingertips. There was Haida Gwaii, the long hard paddle in Hecate Strait (definitely way beyond my comfort zone!) and the long soak in the hot pools, finally after 9 days of camping and no showers. An exquisite luxury. The wild west coast, Flores Island, the beach at Cow Bay, and the beautiful trail through the forest to Ahousaht. And Meares Island, the 1500-year-old trees, gnarled, and bent, looking like the very Form of Ancient.

I remember picking blackberries on the dike by the airport, in the hot sun, stung and raked by thorns. You, always wanting to get just a little more, and me grumbling and reflecting about the line from that song you wrote so many years ago, that summed up your attitude quite well—"'Pick!' cried the vintner." I think of bottling champagne last summer when we were so happily preparing for Tom's wedding. And I think of that earlier time when we bottled it in your mom's basement, the night the Berlin wall came down. It was a particularly explosive mixture. We lost several bottles and it seemed to me somehow appropriate, the champagne flowing, spilling, effusing on the concrete floor, as the Cold War ended. I think of your wine labels, *In vino amor est*, the name conceived many years ago also, and I think that it is not just wine into which you have poured your love. It has gone into so many things—optical systems at Range Vision, photography, the kids, me, our cats, your blog, your revolutionary ideas about the nature of the self (which I try to follow and about which I catch the occasional glimmer of understanding).

You write, "I don't regard the loss of *Gordon Cornwall's* future experiences as a huge loss." Ah, but I do! I think about your whimsy. I know no one else who has that, quite the same way you do. I think about the tree house you built for me in the maple. Remember how I once referred to it as "a canopy viewing platform," upon which Talia exclaimed, "C'mon Mom, we all know it's a tree fort!" I think about your photography, the surreal animals' series, and your newly-developing ability to make people laugh with pictures. I said to you the other day that I thought it had something to do with your reflections about personal identity and you asked me to explain and I tried to make the case, although not very well. But it seems to me that your ideas about the self would naturally enhance your appreciation of the absurd. And is not the absurd a classic ingredient of humor?

If it is really true that we are all under an illusion about the nature of the self, then there is a heck of a lot of illusion around. And yet we are mostly terribly earnest and perhaps even ponderous about ourselves. The Self looms large, and seems solidly rooted. What could be more real? If it should prove to be a will o' wisp, then that is kind of funny. A Cosmic Joke?

You say I shouldn't worry so much or give myself over to imagining doomy possibilities. If you should die, then I will grieve, for sure. I shouldn't grieve now. Why go through it twice? This is rational, but I am not entirely rational. I do not command these visions of the future, although I can suppress them sometimes, will them away. Mostly I do not give myself over to them, although I know that I could. I try to savour the moment—and I do. The ski we had at Callaghan a few weeks ago, the last ski of the season, the snow melting, dissolving, moving towards spring, to awakening and renewal. I enjoyed that. Our trip to Seattle last weekend. Buying you the Raiders of the Lost Ark fedora, appropriate garb perhaps for a dangerous and epic journey. You looking so cool in it, long and lean, and there is something *je ne sais quoi*, about kisses under its sheltering brim. I enjoyed that too. So life is not without its pleasures. The pleasures don't banish the terrors though. It is remarkable how we can live with terrors in our midst. I often think of the airmen of the First and Second World War. The statistics were terribly stacked against those young men—especially in the First World War. They were certainly aware of this, and I marvel that they still went about their business, and did not dissolve into a puddle of anxiety and fear.

You say you will always be with me and it is true, we are so inextricably intertwined. The dead do stay with us. I still think about my father, about his jokes, and the funny (and creative) things he sometimes did. I like retelling my father's jokes and stories, and am pleased that he does live on in this way. But Gordon, it isn't the same! It is a bit of a comfort, but it isn't the same—not one bit! Memories of laughing eyes aren't the same as laughing eyes.

Remember when William died . . . the nurse explained to me that I could have a Caesarian, but in cases like mine, a "natural" delivery was preferable. If I were to become pregnant again, she told me, it was better for *that* baby to be in an intact womb. I agreed to this, and was given oxytocin to start contractions. I don't remember how long it took, a long time, I think. I have no sense of how much time elapsed. One thing I remember was that I didn't cry. Together we walked the halls of the hospital and the baby was eventually born. And when I held him in my arms, the tears came. The nurses told me that they had been worried about me because I hadn't cried and they were relieved that I was finally weeping. They thought that was bet-

ter for my psychological health. I haven't cried at all about the melanoma diagnosis—until now. As I read this over, my eyes well up.

When William died, I grieved, but at the same time, I had hope
that I would have another child. It kept me going. And I was right.
We had two and they have brought us so much joy!

But this! I don't see anything hopeful coming out of it. It is
harder than giving birth to William.

> I love you. I will always love you.
> Claudia

On the 20th, Dr. Zhou phoned Gordon with the results of the PET
scan. We learned that an ominous bright spot was visible. A lymph node
under Gordon's arm "lit" up—glowed yellow and red against a dark-
blue background. The PET scan not only found masses or lumps, it also
revealed metabolic processes indicative of malignant tumors. Since they
grew rapidly, they were energy hogs that absorbed more sugar than
normal tissues did. Before being scanned, Gordon had been injected
with radioactive glucose. The cancer took up this sugar avidly and then
showed up as a luminous speck. A radiologist could easily distinguish it
from benign growths.

Fortunately, Gordon had only one tumor, but the node containing it
and some of the surrounding nodes in his axilla needed to be removed
to prevent further infection. Dr. Zhou proposed the surgery be done at
Lions Gate Hospital in North Vancouver, and Gordon wondered if Dr.
Chang, whom he had already met, could do it. "I'll ask him," said Dr.
Zhou. He also advised Gordon he would continue to follow him with
skin inspections every three months. I was more concerned about the
melanoma assailing Gordon's lungs or other organs. What were we
going to do about that possibility?

The cancer seemed unstoppable. Gordon was just one and a half
months past his original diagnosis and already he was stage III, a milestone I didn't like to consider. But somehow, I kept going. My life still
had a rhythm. Day followed night. I made coffee in the mornings. I fed
our clamoring cat. I critiqued Gordon's latest blogpost. I gave a talk
about my previous book. I had teaching commitments. I went for walks
along the Capilano River. One foot followed the other. Day followed
night.

4

THE MAD RUSH

My fingers scampered over the screen of my iPad. I was playing electronic bridge as we waited to consult Dr. Chang. Whenever I made a contract, I had a feeling of satisfaction—a small mental ping. It alleviated my nervousness, at least momentarily, and helped to pass the time. When Dr. Chang called us in to his office, I felt fairly composed. He gestured to the chairs across from his desk, and Gordon and I sat down to talk about the upcoming lymph node dissection.

Dr. Chang said he would be taking some "double digit" number of nodes out. He explained that he couldn't say exactly how many. It would depend on what he found. He didn't want to take them all; that might cause lymphedema, a swelling in the arm that developed when the lymph nodes were unable to drain properly. "It used to be common after breast cancer surgeries," he said. "But because we are doing fewer mastectomies, we are seeing less of it now." Getting the right number was a balancing act, I gathered. Dr. Chang would take anything that looked infected, but he didn't want to take more than necessary and cause a debilitating side effect either. "I like to think about what could go wrong, so I can prevent it," he said. He also told us that he would remove some more tissue from around the site of Gordon's second melanoma. This was the one that Dr. Zhou had removed in his office, and since it was malignant, protocol dictated an additional excision. Dr. Chang seemed careful and caring; I was pleased he was our surgeon. "I might be able to do this tomorrow, but I only have one operating day a week, so I'll have to check," Dr. Chang explained. Gordon and I were always striving to get medical appointments as soon as possible; still I had no idea you could set up an operation from one day to the next. I was impressed as well as grateful. As it turned out, Dr. Chang was not able to swing this feat, but I thanked him for trying. The dissection was booked for the following week.

> *April 26. Sometimes I feel Gordon's life is hanging by a thread. Would a week earlier make a difference between life and death?*

Ever since Gordon got the diagnosis of melanoma, I had the sense we were in a swirling vortex where things were flying at us from all directions. We could duck one missile, only to be hit with another. I discovered it was not unusual for people like me to feel this way. As Steven Wang wrote:

> There is no doubt that you will go through an intense and stressful period from the time of diagnosis to the time when you complete treatment. I call this period the "mad rush." . . . During treatment, many people feel that the process is chaotic and that they have lost control. Navigating the "mad rush" phase can be challenging, even for many health care professionals.[1]

I was responding to that disagreeable feeling of being out of control, when I asked Gordon to make another appointment with Dr. Zhou. I was convinced the PET scan was an accurate reflection of what was going on and that the pathology report following surgery would find at least one lymph node positive for melanoma. I decided to prepare for this eventuality by securing an appointment with a medical oncologist. I wanted to be able to explore further options as soon as possible after receiving the biopsy.

Removing melanoma surgically (with a wide margin) has been a mainstay of treatment since the early 1900s, but it is a crude instrument.[2] Stray malignant cells can easily escape the surgeon's knife and cause a relapse. So far, we had played catch-up as one lump was removed and then another popped up. I felt the only way to get ahead of the game was with systemic treatment—a drug that could go on the offensive at the cellular level. This approach had done wonders for patients with breast cancer[3] and we had discussed it briefly with the oncologist we had seen. She seemed only able to consider interferon, however, and I thought Dr. Zhou could put us in contact with someone who had more resources. After all, he worked at the headquarters of the BC Cancer Agency in Vancouver—the nerve center of cancer research in the province. We also wanted to ask him about testing Gordon's tumors for the BRAF mutation, as Kathy Barnard had suggested, another preemptive move.

We were unsuccessful on both counts. Dr. Zhou said he didn't know who would pay for the BRAF test. He explained that while drug companies sometimes ordered it in the context of clinical trials, the BC Cancer Agency was not offering it to its patients. I wondered whether we could arrange to cover the fee ourselves, and I made a mental note to investigate. When we asked Dr. Zhou about the referral, he shook his head and said, "No oncologist would see you until we have results of the lymph node dissection." We had to wait for developments. If the melanoma was deemed "unresectable" and surgery considered no longer effective, *then* we could think about cancer drugs and draw on the expertise of a medical oncologist. We left the office feeling flat and frustrated.

> *April 26. All this is distracting me from my work. Neither of us has been sleeping well. The fight or flight emotions are engaged, to very little effect. I should tone them down. If my luck is bad, I live for a matter of months—say the rest of the year. If I stay off toxic chemo, I still might get something useful done with that time although lately, I've found it harder to write and think. If my time frame is that short, I can try to publish short pieces online or try to cobble a book together making liberal use of the work I've already done. But I don't know—my time could be short or long. It's not in my hands.*

Our emotions swung this way and that, from one day to the next, even from one hour to the next. Often we were not in unison.

> *April 28. Gordon feels fine, is cheerful. He sings, whistles, says the future is over-rated.*

I, on the other hand, was hardly ever that light-hearted. So we'd have conversations like this one: "I wish we weren't going through this. Life would be so much nicer if we weren't," I said.

"Life is just fine."

"I'm afraid of losing you!"
"I'm still here!"

April 29. Gordon can feel the lump under his arm now, couldn't seem to before. I just get used to the new normal, "lymph-node involvement," and then there is a newer normal, a palpable lump. I feel the voice of doom is the truth. But I can't tell how useful my emotions are as indicators. They feel unhinged.

Seeking distraction, we went to Lighthouse Park in West Vancouver. On that sleepy Sunday afternoon, the sea was still, trembling a little, under a light breeze. We clambered over rocks and gathered seaweed. I felt a little foolish doing this. I mean who collects seaweed? But I had been reading a new book about edible sea vegetables and was curious. What would they be like? Could we use seaweed to supplement our provisions on kayaking trips? We picked up alaria, sea lettuce, and kelp. We ate some of it raw, and fried some with butter and garlic. The culinary verdict: so-so, but the activity was mildly entertaining.

May 1. Gordon had a good conversation with Kathy Barnard. She said Dr. Smiljanic can get us a BRAF test. She also said there is an ipilimumab trial in Edmonton in which we might be able to participate. (I always say "we." Odd, no?) Kathy somehow takes the terror out of this. But I don't expect the effect to last.

On the morning of May 2, I drove Gordon to Lions Gate Hospital so that he could report for his surgery at ten. I expected to pick him up at about two in the afternoon. By three, I hadn't heard anything. *Somatic symptoms to burn.* I finally got a call near six, telling me I could come.

"Why did it take so long? I asked Gordon, when he got into the car.

He shrugged, "Delays." But nothing to do with his operation, which had lasted about an hour and a half—as predicted. Also as predicted, Dr. Chang had removed a double-digit number of nodes—eighteen to be exact. Gordon was a little sore, but with painkillers, the discomfort was manageable.

May 5. My arm is stapled together in two places like Frankenstein's monster's neck. A disturbing comment post-surgery—the lymph nodes in the vicinity also appeared swollen. I won't know until the path report whether they were infected or not, but I expect they were. They have also been removed. But it seems to me the chances of additional micro-metastases must be high.

May 6. Somewhat rough night. I couldn't sleep.

I was worrying about those enlarged lymph nodes. I found myself troubled by awful, violent images—severed limbs, explosions, axes embedded in my brain. When I told Gordon what was going through my mind, he said, "We have a life-threatening disease to fight, that's all. You don't have to embellish it." This was sensible advice, but not so easy to follow. Psychologists have a name for the phenomenon I was experiencing— "intrusive thoughts." They are disturbing visions of death and injury that are not uncommon in people suffering from extreme anxiety. I felt I was being lashed by a neural storm, but it passed. And then I went back to tackling the melanoma, in itself a frightening enough proposition.

Ten days had gone by since we saw Dr. Zhou. The aura of his certainty—that it was too early for Gordon to see an oncologist—was fading. We decided to talk to Rob about another referral, but this time, we were determined to see Dr. Smiljanic. Rob was in favor of the idea. Later when I reviewed these events with him, he said by way of explanation, "Let me tell you a story."

> I had a patient once to whom I was very close. She got breast cancer so I referred her and she had surgery. The recommendation came back: "We've got it all and you don't need to do anything else." I remember feeling this complete sense of disquiet, but I was younger then and not as confident to go up against the recommendations of the surgeon. So I didn't say anything.
>
> She had a lumpectomy and then she had another lump. And I remember feeling great regret that I had not, even though they had said everything was okay, that I had not pushed for more. Now when I have a patient, I don't care what these guys say, I tell them, "You go flat out."
>
> Let me give you another example. I had a patient who was actually my high school teacher and who got cancer in his fifties. Before he became my patient he was told, "We'll just watch it and observe," and then he became my patient and by that time, the cancer had

spread and he died. He had said to me, "I wish I had been told that this might happen."

I have another patient who came in to me about four or five years ago. He has cancer of the prostate. He was told in a similar vein in his fifties that "Oh, we'll just watch this," and now it's spread. He's very close to his wife and ultimately he's going to die from this.

My point is that when you are faced with a cancer, in my opinion, you need to be as aggressive as you can. When I see something like this, your best chance of a cure is to hit it hard and fast with everything you can at the very beginning.

Some doctors are inclined to be reassuring—telling their patients, "It's nothing," "Not a concern," "Come back in a month if it doesn't clear up." Rob was not one of these—especially when it came to cancer. He asked his assistant to expedite an appointment with Dr. Smiljanic. She worked a miracle and arranged for one in just three days. For the moment, we had done everything we could to push for treatment. But fear and foreboding still had us in its grip. Gordon wrote:

May 8. Dreamt last night that I noticed a litter of kittens in a corner in the bedroom. They were in bad shape, half-dead, many of them extremely emaciated. The closer I looked the more heads I saw—I counted eighteen. Most had no fur on their heads, only skulls, and were eyeless. The best one had a face and a single eye on the right side. In the dream, we made this discovery Saturday night. Tomorrow would be Sunday and the vet would be closed. I was coming to the realization that I'd have to put them out of their misery myself. Strangle them mercifully and bury them in a pit in the garden. When I woke, I figured they were the melanoma.

Or maybe the lymph nodes? After all, there were eighteen of them.

May 10. I am so afraid that we will learn that Gordon's condition is even worse than we expected. Or that there is no possibility of chemo. I feel horrible—cold, heart pounding, stomach churning, dry mouth. I am beside myself.

We arrived at Dr. Smiljanic's office a little early, only to be told that "Sasha" was running late. His office was filled to capacity. Some patients were standing in the hallway outside. After about an hour and a half, the receptionist called Gordon. Dr. Smiljanic was tall, dark-haired, slim, in his forties, I guessed. He shook our hands, sat down, and listened to Gordon's story. When Gordon explained that he was still waiting for the path report on the last surgery, Dr. Smiljanic, said, "Let me look, maybe it's here already." He typed on his keyboard, read something on the monitor, smiled, and swiveled the screen toward us, so we could see too. A small but telling gesture.

The results were better than we anticipated. Only one lymph node contained a tumor—the one that lit up in the PET scan. Some of the others Dr. Chang had removed were enlarged, reacting. But these lymph nodes were not infected. I started to feel better.

Dr. Smiljanic told us that the cancer was quite large, four centimeters in length. Therefore, radiation under Gordon's arm might be in order. Dr. Smiljanic said he would refer Gordon to a radiation oncologist at the BC Cancer Agency to explore that possibility. Cancer cells are especially vulnerable to radiation because they are actively dividing. The therapy has been used for over a hundred years to treat malignancies; we were definitely on familiar ground here. But Gordon also had a question that related to a more recent discovery that Kathy had mentioned—the BRAF mutation. Could his tumors be tested for it? Dr. Smiljanic said he could do this too. If Gordon was positive, he would be in line for Zelboraf, which Health Canada had approved in February 2012.[4] Dr. Smiljanic also said he would try to get ipilimumab.[5] "We don't have much information about these therapies in the adjuvant setting," he admitted. "In five years, we'll know more, but you can't wait that long." I was aware that the drugs had mostly been used to shrink existing tumors. As far as we knew, Gordon didn't *have* any tumors now; the aim of using drugs in the "adjuvant setting" was to destroy malignant cells that might multiply and form lumps. Dr. Smiljanic was telling us that in trying this we would be entering a frontier. I didn't mind that at all; I appreciated his frankness, letting us know that success was uncertain. "I'll give you my e-mail. If you have any concerns, let me know," Dr. Smiljanic said as we got up to go. *His e-mail address*, I thought. *Wow, hardly any doctors give you that.*[6] This unprecedented access quite bowled me over.

Gordon glanced at his watch. He had ten minutes to get to another appointment, a postoperation checkup with Dr. Chang, whose office was just a few blocks away. "I'll have to run," Gordon said. He meant it literally. I laughed when I saw him take off. As I tagged behind at a more leisurely pace, I thought, *It has to be a good sign that he can jog from his oncologist to his surgeon.* I was also pleased by how much Gordon's prospects had improved in a mere fifteen minutes. The BRAF test was not a problem, after all. And there were things we could do to try to prevent recurrence. We didn't have to wait for the melanoma to rear up again. Maybe best of all, Dr. Smiljanic indicated he was willing to try for some of the newer therapies. On May 10, Dr. Smiljanic wrote a letter to Rob to keep him abreast of what was happening: "Gordon is going to go to the Cancer Agency for an opinion [about radiation], while I work on some form of adjuvant therapy for him. Interferon would be next to useless, hopefully we can come up with something more innovative."

We were suddenly on a much more positive path.

5

DON'T WORRY ABOUT IT

On the long May weekend, we drove to our cabin at Sheridan Lake in the Cariboo—three hundred miles north of Vancouver, on a plateau, four thousand feet above sea level, cattle ranching country, something of an economic backwater. Gordon has been coming up ever since he was ten, when his mother and a friend of hers bought the property, and I started visiting when I was seventeen. We know the place in all its seasons—we swim and canoe in the summer, ski over the ice in winter and early spring. The cabin is off the grid. No cell phone coverage, no hydro-supplied electricity. A small solar panel powers a couple of lights; we have a coal and wood stove for heating and cooking, a pump for drawing water from the lake. The place has been good to us, a refuge. We slow down when we get there, sleep more than usual—because of the altitude we say.

We arrived on Friday, and the next morning Talia and her boyfriend, Pat, joined us. We cooked, watched the loons and geese fight over the nesting real estate, listened to the trees sighing in the wind, went for a walk, played bridge, and talked. But it wasn't going to be a normal restful weekend. On Saturday night, when we had gone to bed, I asked Gordon how he was:

"Okay."

But I detected hesitation. "Is something wrong?"

"I'm worried about my arm. There's another lump."

I felt sick. I was sleepy when we went to bed. Suddenly all thought of sleep was gone. I was staring at the shadowy walls, wide-eyed. "When did you notice it?"

"Just now when I went to bed."

"We better go home early."

"Yeah," said Gordon.

On Sunday, when I opened my diary, my receptacle for grim thoughts, I wrote:

> *May. 20. The implacable march of the melanoma. Gordon has had five surgeries so far. The first lump twice, the second lump twice, the lymph nodes and now this. Five surgeries since February. It is only May.*

Gordon and I left sooner than we'd planned, on the holiday Monday, so that we could deal with the new development as soon as possible. We took what we call "the back way," through the hamlets of Clinton, and Lillooet, along Seton Lake and tumbling Cayoosh Creek, past Duffy Lake, the glacier-ringed Joffre Lakes, through the Mount Currie Native Reserve and some more small towns, Pemberton and Whistler, then past Black Tusk, a thumb-like extrusion of volcanic rock, along Howe Sound and home. The scenery was spectacular, but I hardly noticed.

First thing on Tuesday, Gordon called Dr. Chang's office for an appointment. He got one for the same day—at noon. I always hated waiting; it made me feel like we were in a dead zone. All I could do was stew; I found it difficult to concentrate on anything else. I was glad to see us moving along in this way. Then Gordon told me Dr. Chang had ordered an investigative ultrasound for later that afternoon and I began to feel even happier. We were traveling at a good clip indeed! But I was dashed when Gordon came home after the scan. He said, "The technician operating the ultrasound thinks there's a problem. He's going to fax the results to Dr. Chang." At five o'clock, the end of his day, Dr. Chang phoned. He explained, "The lump is a seroma—a pocket of clear fluid that sometimes forms after surgery. We can drain it and I'll order a biopsy to make certain." I was relieved, although the emotional roller coaster took its toll. I wrote: *I am exhausted.*

*June 8. I had a dream. There was a cubby hole in our bedroom. In it,
a snake, about half the circumference of my arm, lay coiled. It was a
cubby like those in the zoo, but no glass between the snake and us. I
was worried about the snake, didn't know whether it was poisonous
or not.*

The dream echoed my waking fears—of an uncertain hazard near to us
and from which we were not shielded.

The new mass was not an issue, but Gordon and I were still eager to
find a treatment that might prevent more tumors from forming. Dr.
Smiljanic had explained that not much was known about ipilimumab's
ability to prevent relapse but that the therapy was still worth trying.
Indeed, I found some results from a recent study that, though small,
supported his opinion. In Florida, a team of researchers gave seventy-
five individuals ipilimumab following surgery for melanoma. With the
drug, 40 percent of stage IV patients were disease-free after five years,
and a higher proportion—65 percent—of stage III patients were. For
both groups, the results were significantly better than what you could
expect from surgery alone. The investigators termed the work "promising" and called for a larger trial to confirm the findings.[1] We didn't have
a lot to go on, but here was some evidence that ipilimumab could
improve Gordon's chances. The data were also an argument for obtaining the drug sooner (at stage III) rather than later.

The BC Cancer Agency had still not decided to fund ipilimumab, so
Dr. Smiljanic applied directly to its developer, Bristol-Myers Squibb, to
ask for the drug on compassionate grounds. But I knew that impedi-
ments could arise. The story of Darcy Doherty, running through the
media at the time, was proof of that. He was a forty-eight-year-old
Canadian, a father of three who was dying of metastatic melanoma. It
had spread to his brain, which meant his condition was critical. Doherty
and his physician thought that nivolumab, a drug BMS was currently
investigating but which was not approved for general use, might save his
life. He was ineligible for clinical trials then available; they excluded
patients with brain metastases. Doherty hoped BMS would give him
nivolumab through a compassionate care program, which usually has
more generous rules. However, the company refused. BMS maintained
the medicine wasn't yet safe to use outside a clinical trial—a decision
Doherty and his family had difficulty comprehending. How could side

effects of nivolumab make Doherty any worse than he already was? Another factor may also have been at play. Later when I talked to Tim Turnham, executive director of the Melanoma Research Foundation in Washington, D.C., he explained:

> The companies don't put a compassionate program in place until they have done their clinical trials. Often, their philosophy is that the best thing for the biggest group of patients is to get good, effective drugs on the market as quickly and cleanly as possible. If they open up a lot of these expanded access, compassionate use protocols, the data and information get cluttered. If you have a compassionate use program, and all of a sudden two people die on that program, that could slow down or jeopardize the entire drug approval process. Then people might begin to say, "Well let's slow down the approval and take a look and understand this."

By July 10, 2012, almost 200,000 of Doherty's supporters had signed a Change.org petition pleading his case, but BMS didn't budge.[2] Doherty died a month later.

Drug companies are not legally obliged to provide compassionate relief, and you certainly couldn't count on them to do it. I decided it might be prudent to explore a back-up plan. While Dr. Smiljanic was looking into compassionate care, I searched for a clinical trial. Kathy had mentioned that Dr. Michael Smylie was starting to recruit patients for an ipilimumab study at the Cross Cancer Institute in Edmonton, and I wondered if Gordon could participate. When I phoned Dr. Smylie's office, his clinical trials assistant, Shelley, took my call. After I related Gordon's story, she said he sounded like a good candidate; we should hear back soon.

To be accepted in the trial, Gordon needed to meet a set of strict criteria. Researchers at BMS had designed the experiment to answer a specific set of questions, and only those people who could help them get the answers they needed would be enrolled. Being able to benefit from the drug was not by itself a reason to be accepted. Patients who did not fit the terms of the study would miss out on a potentially life-saving medicine. I knew that whether Gordon would be allowed in was unclear. I also realized that even if Gordon enrolled in the trial and received the new therapy, he might not respond. This was a voyage into the unknown.

A few days after my conversation with Shelley, Gordon and I sat in the bowels of the BC Cancer Agency—in a small beige windowless room with no distracting or comforting elements. We had come to talk to Dr. Charmaine Kim-Sing about radiation. Gordon told her that Dr. Smiljanic was looking into a systemic drug treatment for him but wondered whether radiation should come first. Dr. Kim-Sing had a wealth of information at her fingertips and spoke to us in the authoritative manner of a university professor, which she also was. She gave us many numbers to consider. She said radiation carried a 30 percent risk of long-term lymphedema, the swelling caused when the lymph nodes are unable to drain properly, and would damage 20 percent of Gordon's left lung—probably permanently. Gordon's skin would become red and sore, an effect that might actually get worse for one or two weeks after the treatment ended. Radiation would hold up any drug infusions Gordon might be contemplating. It would take two to three weeks to finish the preparations. The radiation itself would be delivered in twenty daily doses (or fractions) over a period of four weeks. Then Gordon would need to recover for four weeks before he could start another therapy, so the delay would amount to at least ten or eleven weeks. The risk of local recurrence would drop from 25 percent to 6 percent. Paradoxically, a statistical analysis showed the treatment did not lead to an improvement in life expectancy—that is, a 0 percent gain. Dr. Kim-Sing told us that she was relying on research out of Australia, a country where physicians had much experience with melanoma.

We headed back to North Vancouver. I didn't say anything, at first. I was trying to digest the disappointing results of our discussion. But as we were crossing the Cambie Street viaduct, I had an idea. I turned to Gordon, who was driving, and said, "If there is no survival benefit to radiation, why does anybody bother doing it? The side effects aren't trivial."

"I had the same thought," Gordon said. "Maybe it's not worth doing."

"Or maybe," I said, "there are other opinions about the survival benefit. I'm going to look into it."

When we got home, Gordon e-mailed Dr. Smiljanic. "Today I saw Dr. Charmaine Kim-Sing. She gave what I thought was a clear and thorough briefing on the risks and benefits of local radiation therapy in my axillary area. Dr. Kim-Sing did not recommend radiation treatment, nor did she recommend against it, but left the decision in my hands." Gordon also wrote, "I don't clearly understand *why* radiation therapy has no long-term survival benefit." Dr. Smiljanic replied at length by e-mail that evening:

> The lack of long term survival has to do with our historical inability to find any useful drugs for melanoma. Simply put, who cares if we radiate the armpit to prevent a relapse in this area when the disease just pops up in the liver and lungs. For local treatments (radiation to a specific area) to be beneficial, it is my opinion that they need to be coupled with systemic (ipi) treatments that cut down the risk of metastasis. This is a key point. . . . ALL DATA POINTING TO A LACK OF SURVIVAL FOR AXILLARY RADIATION IS DE-RIVED FROM PRE IPI AND ZELBORAF DATA [Dr. Smiljanic's emphasis]. In other words, I am no longer sure that radiation is ineffective when we have better tools such as ipi and emerging agents.
>
> The primary goal should be the ipi. I would speak to the ipi study nurses [in Edmonton] to carefully clarify what is allowed in terms of radiation. You may be excluded from the trial if you have radiation, you also may be allowed to do radiation DURING the ipi (as has been done many times with brain metastasis). If the radiation in any way jeopardizes your ability to access ipi then forgo it.

While Dr. Smiljanic put the priority on ipilimumab, he also told Gordon that combining it with radiation could have even better results. In the same e-mail, he mentioned a new report from some researchers at Stanford University. It showed that radiation and ipilimumab appeared to be synergistic in the treatment of melanoma. Radiation seemed to increase the antitumor effect of the drug.[3] The paper caused a flurry of interest in the oncology world, and further studies of the phenomenon were likely to follow. "Radiation," Dr. Smiljanic wrote, "might have an important but 'undefined' role."

I began trolling the Internet to learn more. Dr. Kim-Sing was correct in telling us that radiation tended to prevent local recurrence. She was also right that you could find a body of research showing it did not improve overall life expectancy.[4] However, on the Alberta Health Services website, I found an alternative point of view. Here a discussion cited a 2009 paper about the benefits of radiation in a study of 615 melanoma patients who had lymph node surgery. Of those who didn't have radiation, 30 percent were alive five years after their operation. On the other hand, 55 percent of the patients who had radiation were going strong at five years.[5]

Gordon termed the confusion in which we found ourselves "the fog of medicine."[6] He was alluding to an idea made famous by German military theorist Carl von Clausewitz, who wrote in his book *On War*, "Lastly, the great uncertainty of all data in War is a peculiar difficulty, because all action must, to a certain extent, be planned in a mere twilight, which in addition not unfrequently—like the effect of a fog or moonshine—gives to things exaggerated dimensions and an unnatural appearance."[7] Modern medical theorists have pointed out that physicians, like soldiers, also have to make choices in conditions of uncertainty. Benjamin Djulbegovic, a professor of medicine at the University of South Florida, advises, "Clausewitz . . . believed that action should remain in the hands of the capable commander in the field whose creativity, talent, and genius will be able to guide his troops through the fog of the battle. Likewise, decisions for individual patients will always remain with skilful doctors able to navigate successfully through the sea of uncertainty of clinical practice."[8]

According to Clausewitz, the important question was "Who can we trust?" not "What can we trust?" But that one was not so easy to answer either. I was inclined to look at both questions. Dr. Smiljanic had written to Gordon about the changing landscape of melanoma treatment due to the discovery of new immunotherapies. I respected his clinical judgment and experience. When you combined that with what I had found—a study showing benefits for radiation even without immunotherapy—the case for radiation started to look more attractive. I knew we couldn't snap our fingers and cure Gordon's melanoma. But we could look for ways to give him an edge.

We were still mulling over this option when we heard from Shelley in Edmonton. We were out of luck. As Gordon relayed to Dr. Smiljanic in an e-mail, "I am now told I do not qualify, because no tumor is known to remain in my body. The focus of the trial is on cure of known disease, not adjuvant. If I had another scan which revealed a tumor, I would then qualify." Since it seemed that Gordon was ineligible for the trial, he had questions for Dr. Smiljanic: "I understand Health Canada guidelines indicate that ipi is a second-line treatment to be used only if another drug has failed. Is there any flexibility there? If the ipi door is closed (for now), do you think I should have the RT? (Some studies do show survival benefits.)"

Later that evening Dr. Smiljanic replied. He told Gordon that there was no flexibility about the Health Canada requirements—he had to have old-style chemo first.[9] Dr. Smiljanic explained, "We have had to do this with every ipi patient we have treated over the last 2 years." He also clarified that the ipi door wasn't really closed. "Just the trial is closed . . . we are going to push BMS to let us use the drug for you. And yes, I would still do the radiation if it were me."

Gordon followed this advice. Since the ipilimumab trial in Edmonton was not a go, he was most likely to get the drug through Dr. Smiljanic after all. He expected it would take several months to obtain, allowing him to have radiation and recover. He was now willing to risk the negative side effects of the treatment because he believed it might have benefits overall. So on June 22, Gordon went to the cancer agency for planning, a scan, and mold making. The mold would be used to create a plaster cast, which would hold Gordon's shoulder firmly in place and allow the radiation beams to be directed at the appropriate area under Gordon's arm.

We were in a race with a swift competitor who often left us sputtering in the dust. And so it was again. The melanoma burst ahead. The day after Gordon visited the cancer agency, he discovered yet another lump—in his left armpit. He wrote in his blog, "The lump was small, like a dried lentil that moved under my skin when I felt it."[10] He e-mailed Dr. Smiljanic about it, who responded immediately. He thought it was "unlikely" that a new tumor would have emerged so soon after the surgery—although it was "possible." He suggested that Gordon let Dr. Kim-Sing have a look at it.

Gordon recalled how he was wrong about the previous lump. He wrote, "I knew my self-diagnostics were fallible, and I was at risk of being labeled a hypochondriac."[11] Nevertheless, he reported his discovery to Dr. Kim-Sing's office. Her assistant called back with a message from Dr. Kim-Sing. "It's probably just scar tissue or another seroma. Don't worry about it."[12]

But the lump continued to grow. "This was no time to save face,"[13] Gordon decided. He thought a professional should at least have a look at it, and he visited Rob, who was able to fit him in at short notice. Rob said it felt like a tumor. Gordon called Dr. Kim-Sing again—now with the information that his GP thought the lump was a tumor. This time she suggested Gordon see Dr. Chang. If Gordon did have a melanoma, Dr. Chang would have to remove it before she could begin her treatment. She told Gordon she would put the radiation on hold in case he had another cancer. She asked to be posted on events, which Gordon promised to do.

We were in the middle of a maelstrom. Remarkably, Gordon was still managing to think about *The Phantom Self*. On the morning of June 28 he wrote in his journal:

Who am I?
Someone in the past who led me here.
Someone whose future is in my hands.
Who am I?
Anyone who pointed me in this direction.
Anyone whose life I will affect or can touch.

In the afternoon, Gordon went to see Dr. Chang, who had kindly agreed to examine him. Later Gordon wrote in his blog: "To expedite the diagnosis, he offered to attempt a needle biopsy there in the office; but the effort was unsuccessful; the lump was hard to hit with the needle, because it was too mobile, because of its awkward location in my armpit, and because he had to do it 'blind,' working without imaging technology."[14] Dr. Chang ordered an ultrasound with a needle biopsy at Lions Gate Hospital. But Gordon and I knew it could take weeks before we had an answer. If the news was bad and the pathology indicated melanoma, we'd have to wait—for a surgery date. And then we'd have to wait again—for Gordon to heal—before he could finally embark on the radiation that might prevent more of these lumps. These delays would just give comfort to the enemy—allow the melanoma to spread.

A PET scan would give us answers directly. But the BC Cancer Agency was unlikely to order a second scan just six weeks after the first. It metes them out fairly parsimoniously because we have only two such machines in BC—one at the BC Cancer Agency and one at a private clinic in Burnaby.[15] When I phoned the private clinic I discovered it was closed for maintenance, so I rang up the Swedish Medical Center in Seattle. Founded by a Swedish doctor in 1910, it is now the largest nonprofit health-care provider in the Seattle area and offers a variety of services—cardiology, oncology, neurology, radiology. I said my husband needed a PET scan and I explained that we didn't have American insurance but would be paying for the imaging ourselves.

"When would you like to come in?" I was asked.

"When can you do it?"

"Let me check," the receptionist said, and then I heard, "Would Monday work for you?" It was Thursday, so this was just one working day away. I didn't expect Gordon would get in that promptly, so I asked, "Do you mean this coming Monday?"

"Yes," she said.

Then the receptionist told me all we needed to complete the arrangements was a referral from one of our physicians. Gordon visited our long-suffering GP and explained what he was trying to do. Rob, who is usually quite efficient, faxed off the requisition right away, and Gordon was booked in for Monday. Gordon was pleased with what we had achieved but also a little uneasy: Being treated as a customer had its benefits. You got what you wanted when you wanted it. However, buying health care wasn't exactly like buying an appliance or a suit of clothes. Determining what you needed was harder; the customer wasn't always right. Gordon wrote:

> June 30. This gets us into an uncomfortable level of micromanagement of my health care. But it seems necessary to be that proactive. My melanoma is so aggressive! The risk is that we'll blunder. It's important to play it very smart, and not get carried away by emotion. I am handling it okay, I think, but have noticed some lapses—forgot my hat at Chang's; forgot my iPad and a letter at Scott's. Claudia is okay for the most part but sometimes becomes unduly mournful.

We drove down to the U.S. border on July 2, a warm sunny day. Despite the fine weather, traffic was light and only a few cars were lined up at the crossing. When the American official asked us what the purpose of our visit was, Gordon said, "It's for a PET scan." The guard asked, "So where's the pet?" We were puzzled a moment; then we realized he was making a joke.

After barreling south along the I-5 highway for a couple of hours, we arrived at the Swedish Medical Center in downtown Seattle. A receptionist greeted us warmly and directed us to the accounting department. The total cost of the scan was $5,050 (US). Since Gordon was paying immediately (with a credit card), he was given a 35 percent discount. As any savvy consumer knows, many prices are not set in stone. We didn't realize that the cost of medical care was negotiable in the United States. Later we learned that because the American multi-payer insurance system is so baroque for clinics and hospitals to navigate, deductions for paying on the spot are not uncommon.[16] The discovery was a pleasant surprise.

When the scan was over, a technician gave Gordon a disc containing the results and said a radiologist would fax him a report the next day. We drove back north, taking the scenic route along the coast, the Chuckanut Drive. For dinner, we stopped at the Oyster Bar, one of our favorite restaurants. A small establishment located on a steep bank close to the water, it offers views of the San Juan Islands. As we sat down at our table, the waiter noticed that Gordon was wearing a button reading "Stop Coal." "What's that about?" he wanted to know. Gordon explained that in May we had joined a protest in White Rock, a small town very close to the American-Canadian border. We were concerned about the coal trains coming up from the United States to Roberts Bank in Canada. The waiter nodded and gestured to the railway tracks visible on the shore below the restaurant. He said, "That's where the train goes. They use open cars and coal dust blows up from the track. It's not healthy at all." I was startled to run into an eco friendly person and I smiled. *You never know where you might encounter a Green*, I thought while we ate our oysters washed down with a local Sauvignon Blanc.

As promised, we got the report on Tuesday. It clattered through our ancient fax machine at 2:30 in the afternoon. There was a single nodule in the left axilla "most likely representing metastatic disease." Gordon's suspicions were confirmed. He had mixed feelings about this. "On the one hand, it was bad news—another tumor. On the other hand, I now met the criteria for the Edmonton ipi trial."[17] We were in strange territory, where bad news was good news and you had to get worse to have a prospect of getting better.

The next day, our son, Tom, called. He had sustained a concussion playing soccer. *First Gordon and now Tom!* I wanted to scream, but I didn't.

"I feel okay, Mom, Tom said. "I'm going out to UBC today for a meeting."

"Do you think that's wise?"

"I'll be fine."

I tried not to worry, but, of course I did.

On July 4, Gordon called Shelley to see whether he could now enroll in the Edmonton trial. For a second time, she had to let him down. In the space of a week, the study had become full. It could not accept another patient. The experiment was part of an international research project following seven hundred individuals worldwide and originally, the sponsor, Bristol-Myers Squibb, expected it would take a year or more to find them all. However, the recruitment was complete in four weeks. The trial was closed, not just in Edmonton, but in every center running it. *Is there a melanoma epidemic?* Gordon wondered.

Every year, the number of melanoma cases worldwide increases—at a rate much faster than is seen with any other cancer.[18] The malignancy is also one of the most deadly. As Teresa Petrella, an oncologist at the Odette Center in Toronto, writes, "The prognosis for patients with metastatic melanoma is quite dismal as the disease is almost invariably incurable."[19] Customary treatments have not been effective. Therefore, she explains: "The current standard of care for metastatic melanoma in Canada is clinical trials."[20] This put enormous pressure on those experiments; patients knew they were their best chance. Shelley's phone call brought it home to us—finding a spot in a study wasn't going to be easy; these slots were a scarce commodity. Even if you met the conditions of a trial, you might not be accepted. Gordon was in competition with other melanoma patients, and they with him. If he got in somewhere, maybe someone else, perhaps equally deserving, equally beloved, was out in the cold. It was an uncomfortable situation. In our society, we are used to inequality. Not everyone gets the same size slice of pie. Yet everyone usually gets something. Here, though, it was all or nothing. "In the face of limited resources and unlimited demand, every society must eventually confront the ethical dilemmas of health care rationing,"[21] writes Reshma Jagsi, an assistant professor of medicine who researches bioethical issues at the University of Michigan. Options are stark especially when it comes to clinical trials. Access to them is even more restricted than it is to treatment. And yes, moral issues do arise. But I pushed them aside; my biggest concern was finding effective treatment for Gordon.

"Back to Plan A," Gordon wrote. "Surgery followed by radiation."[22] On Friday, we saw Dr. Chang, who shook his head when we told him what had happened: "I don't think you should have had to pay for that scan yourself." Both Gordon and I shrugged. What else could we do? Dr. Chang scheduled Gordon for an operation four days later, on Tuesday. Gordon then called Dr. Kim-Sing's office to give her an update. Later she told me in a phone interview that when she heard the news, her heart sank and she thought, *It doesn't look good at all.* She wrote to Rob: "This man's melanoma is behaving in a very aggressive fashion and is particularly worrisome."[23] She also explained that Gordon was still going ahead with the radiation treatment, but a little later than original-ly planned—on July 16.

Did our efforts to expedite matters really help? Did removing this particular cancer two or three weeks earlier change the outcome for Gordon? It's probably impossible to say. In general, speeding up proce-dures and appointments was the right call, and our disposition to do that probably served us in good stead. Melanoma can go from nothing to stage IV in less than six months. As Dr. Steven Wang observes in his book about melanoma, "You need to take action and take action fast. Certainly, your physician will urge you to undergo treatments as soon as possible—and this urgency is necessary."[24]

We were contending with a formidably difficult disease. "I'm en-gaged in a life-or-death struggle,"[25] Gordon wrote. We were also trying to make the medical system work for us; it was a complex service that had to respond to many people's urgent needs, not just ours. Its practi-tioners were mostly well intentioned, though fallible and under pres-sure. How could we navigate the shoals? Find the safest channels? I reminded myself that we did have resources. Medical knowledge had evolved and innovative pharmaceuticals were available (though not al-ways easy to come by). Gordon and I were also a good team. Whereas I was excitable and alert to problems, Gordon tended not to worry and to be more deliberate. He thought his ideas about the nature of the self helped him to stay calm and reasonable. In his blog, he wrote:

> I can only report that—compared to other times in my life when a lot has been at stake—I feel less anxious. That is worth something. I am less obsessed with my own future than I used to be, and more engaged with other people. All animals—all vertebrates, at least—are jolted into action by the "fight-or-flight" emotions when an obvious threat to survival appears on the present scene. The human animal has a uniquely well-developed ability to project those emotions onto threats which are merely imagined. We are easily panicked by dangers that are not clear and present—that are far off, sometimes predictable, often very uncertain. The fight-or-flight emotions are well adapted for fighting and fleeing, not for long-term planning. They provide motivation, but do not channel it effectively into the intricately coordinated actions required to accomplish long-term plans.
>
> Finding the least-hazardous path through the smoke and hubbub requires sensitive discernment and good judgement—abilities easily overwhelmed by primal emotion. As I search, I am, I admit, looking out for Gordon. But I am moved more by sympathy, and by shared goals, than by self-concern, and I think that makes me more effective. It certainly makes the journey pleasanter.[26]

Gordon was not so susceptible to the hot emotions, the fierce interest we take in our own futures. He wasn't indifferent to what might happen to him; but he wasn't consumed by it. I, on the other hand, was very subject to those emotions. They swept over me like a great tide.

July 10. Surgery day. I am feeling the enormity of possible loss.

Nevertheless, fear (as Gordon also observes) can be useful. I was able to move on a dime—appraise a situation and act accordingly. We were the yin and the yang; hot and cool, fast and steadfast, light and dark. We complemented each other. Together we were much stronger than the sum of our two selves.

6

WE HAVE NO WAY OF MONITORING SUCCESS

To preserve our sanity, we were always trying to carve out periods when we wouldn't be doing anything related to melanoma. The weekend before Gordon started radiation, we went to Galiano Island. A short ferry ride away from the mainland, it has a microclimate of its own—drier and sunnier than our coast. We meandered along the seashore over mossy outcroppings and through sun-strewn arbutus groves. We walked out to Dionisio Point and had a picnic lunch overlooking Georgia Strait. But when we returned to the cottage where we were staying, thoughts encroached. Cancer is like that—it *trespasses*. I complained in my diary: *Wish I didn't have this emptiness—this shadow accompanying me. I carry this image—life without Gordon. What would it be like? What are all the myriad ways I would miss him? I told Gordon what I was thinking, and he said, "Don't make a ghost of me!"*

But Gordon, too, was wrestling with dark apprehensions:

> *July 14. I'm spooked by the thought that the melanoma could have metastasized to my brain—as it sometimes does—and that tumors are growing there, unfelt by me and undetected by the PET/CT scans I've had. Smiljanic says PET scans can't see brain tumors because the brain is such a good absorber of sugar that the whole thing lights up like a tumor! Another kind of scan is needed which he would order prior to my chemo or ipi treatment.*

On July 16, we were back in town, and in the afternoon Gordon drove over to the BC Cancer Agency, found the radiation department, and climbed onto a narrow scanning bed. He lay down, tucked his shoulder into a cradle made to hold it firmly in place, and stared up at the radiotherapy machine. His chest had been tattooed with a black mark, the size of a pinprick, to guide it. Peel-off plastic labels affixed to his skin assisted with alignment. A nurse deftly adjusted the placement of Gordon's shoulder so that the radiation would hit him according to plan. She left the room and high-energy X-rays struck Gordon's axilla, first from above and then from below. The machine buzzed briefly while it was on and then went silent; the therapy was over in about a minute. Gordon was slated for twenty days of treatment, so it was one down and nineteen to go.

On day three I wrote:

July 19. Gordon is not fatigued or sore.

This was good, of course, but at the same time, our son, Tom, had begun to develop debilitating symptoms from his concussion: vertigo, light sensitivity, noise sensitivity, fatigue, sleep disturbance, and some memory problems. He wore a toque even though it was summer and stayed inside with the curtains drawn. He found computers difficult to use; screens made him nauseous. He stopped going to university. I added Tom to my long list of concerns and I told Gordon, "I think I'm being punished." He said, "That's crazy talk." I knew it didn't make any sense, but still that's the way I felt.

To leave the mornings free for writing, Gordon had requested that his radiation appointments be in the afternoon. He was filling notebooks with pages of his small and occasionally indecipherable script. His enthusiasm for the subject was undampened:

July 22. If I am right, then we are strongly inclined by nature not to believe the truth about ourselves, but its opposite. The simple truth is that the relationships that connect us to ourselves, at different times, are not fundamentally different from the relationships that connect us to other people. There is no privileged connection that can justify anticipating our own experience in the future and no one else's—no connection that justifies the motivational force which we allow our anticipated future to have on us.

Gordon didn't think we should neglect ourselves but that the "motivational force" prompting us to work on our own behalf was too strong. We had an unjustified bias and expended too much effort on ourselves at the expense of other people. Incongruously, while Gordon was writing this, he was in a situation in which he suddenly had to spend much more energy than usual looking after himself. His body's claims for attention could not easily be brushed aside. Toward the end of the first week of radiation, Gordon noticed a burning sensation when urinating and also low-level fever and chills. The burning went away, but the fever did not. He knew it could be an effect of the radiation, that it wasn't unusual.

But two weeks into the radiotherapy, early on a Sunday, Gordon woke up feeling distinctly unwell. The fever was much worse. Shivery, he couldn't get warm even though he put on a sweater as well as a fleece jacket. Rob's office was closed and I thought a walk-in clinic wouldn't have the resources to sort out the situation. I drove Gordon through the deserted streets to Lions Gate Hospital. The emergency department was quiet and he didn't wait long to be seen. He related his saga to Dr. Bruce Long, the physician on duty—the skirmishes with lumps, the surgeries, the radiation barrage. Dr. Long ordered a battery of tests—full blood work (seven vials), a chest X-ray, prostate exam, urinalysis. After several hours, he came back with a verdict. Smiling, he said, "You're not worrying me anymore. You have a urinary tract infection. You need antibiotics." All the other test results were good. Gordon started on Cipro right away and felt markedly better after the first tablet.

That night, I had a dream. In it I said, "Gordon has melanoma, Tom has a concussion, and now I'm five months pregnant and I haven't been to the doctor yet!" I was long past the age where an unwanted pregnancy was a concern, but the dream was expressing that sense I had of things piling on. Just when I thought I had enough problems, something else happened. Cancer did not make you invulnerable to other ills.

Aug 1. A beautiful day; I feel tight as a wire.

In the afternoon, Gordon saw Dr. Smiljanic, who told him that he would probably get ipilimumab from BMS on compassionate grounds. Though Gordon's acceptance into the program was not finalized, this was definitely encouraging. Provided things went according to plan, BMS would supply the drug and pay for it, until the BC Cancer Agency funded the therapy. Although BMS normally charged $30,000 per infusion, how much each dose cost the drug maker was a closely guarded secret. I didn't know exactly what BMS would be spending to get Gordon (and other patients) the therapy they required. Even so, the fact that the company seemed willing to provide this assistance was changing my opinion of Big Pharma. Perhaps these corporations weren't as heartless as I was inclined to think. Dr. Smiljanic told us that, ironically, once the BC Cancer Agency decided to foot the bill for the new immunotherapy, some patients might have more difficulty accessing it. They would have to fit the agency's criteria, which could be less inclusive than the drug company's.

As we knew from Gordon's e-mail correspondence with Dr. Smiljanic, he needed to meet Health Canada guidelines about taking ipilimumab as a second line of defense. Dr. Smiljanic picked an older systemic treatment for him to try first—dacarbazine. Used to treat melanoma for the last thirty years, it targets cells that divide and multiply rapidly. But the drug achieves a complete remission in just 5 percent of melanoma patients and a mere quarter of those stay cancer-free.[1] The chemotherapy is chemically related to mustard gas used in the First World War, so perhaps it is no wonder that it has toxic effects—low white blood cell count, an increased risk of infections, nausea, vomiting, loss of appetite, fatigue, headaches, muscle aches, and fever. The fact that it has been approved for so long is a testament to the utter dearth of options. I even wondered whether a placebo would be better. At least it wouldn't make Gordon feel sick.

So why should Gordon start with something that had such a dismal record? Had Health Canada designated ipilimumab as a second line of defense rather than first line because of the cost? When I asked Eric Morrisette, a senior media relations officer with Health Canada, about this, he replied by e-mail that "the only thing Health Canada looks at is whether the drug is safe, efficacious, and of suitable quality." This didn't really explain why a therapy would be designated second line rather than first line. In any case, I realized we could do nothing to change the system—the complex intersection of protocols and directives that governed both patients and physicians. Gordon had to follow the rules. After completing radiation, he would get dacarbazine.

> *August 7. I have a hard time knowing what attitude to take to the future. Gordon appears quite healthy. The fever, chills and fatigue he had in the second week of radiation are gone. Yesterday, he mowed the lawn and then trimmed the laurel hedge and cooked the pork ribs we took over to Tom and Leanna's. So if you didn't know about the melanoma, you would suspect nothing.*

Gordon finished his course of radiation without further incident. On August 10, a CT scan of his head was negative for a brain tumor, dispelling some of our fears—temporarily. In a fairly positive frame of mind, we left for the cottage— just the two of us and our cat, Charlie. Gordon wanted to rest and heal before his chemo treatment.

After weeks of warm sunny weather, the lake temperature was a seductive 70 degrees. We swam several times a day in the silken water—usually out to The Rock, our favorite destination, about 75 meters offshore. Gordon had been cautioned about swimming in "wild" water, for fear of catching an infection, but he couldn't resist. Anyway, he thought he wasn't nearly as likely to catch something swimming in the lake as in a public pool. As usual, we lingered over breakfast, slept a lot; and Gordon chopped wood. We also worked on a video—a short film the organizers of the conference in San Rafael asked to have for their website.

With his camera, Gordon catches Charlie stalking a mouse. He is slinking silently and deliberately under the front deck of our cabin—on the hunt. Intent, his eyes do not leave the quarry. In the voice-over, Gordon explains that Charlie has a 3-D self-model that guides his movement through the world. It keeps him out of trouble and helps him achieve his goals. Suddenly Charlie pounces and Gordon pans discreetly away.

At this point, I take over the camera and focus on Gordon, who is standing in front of a bank of trees. He explains that human beings also have 3-D models but, unlike Charlie, they are interested in what happens at times and places far removed from the present. "This is key to understanding what makes humans tick," Gordon says. "It made one unimpressive primate species into the alpha species that transformed its entire planet." We won "the evolutionary arms race" but at a cost. We strive toward far distant goals and carry out complex plans, but we fret inordinately about our personal futures. Gordon says that caring about what happens to ourselves does not feel optional, in a way in which caring about others does. We feel compelled to think like this, but in fact, Gordon maintains, we are under an illusion, which he pledges to explicate. The video is a teaser, made to intrigue. Gordon leaves the full explanation for the conference. The late afternoon sun plays over Gordon's face; loons call in the distance. I wonder whether he can really make his case. The arguments are difficult, haunting like the calls of loons.

Just when we began to unwind a little, we were reminded of our situation. Another lump emerged—the sixth one—under Gordon's arm where the lymph nodes were excised. It was larger than the others—the size of a golf ball—and it oozed. Gordon suspected it was an artifact of his recent therapy. But to be sure, he made an appointment to consult a radiologist at the cancer agency, once we were back in North Vancouver.

"I hope it's not a melanoma," I said.

"A melanoma doesn't ooze," Gordon said.

"It could be both—an infection and a melanoma."

"You don't have to imagine the worst possible outcome. What about adding a thermonuclear bomb and an earthquake?"

Dr. Kim-Sing was away on holiday so when Gordon got home he saw another radiologist. After Gordon recounted his story, the doctor examined him. He told Gordon the lump was a seroma, not a concern, and said the radiation nurses could instruct him about treating the ooziness. He also made some disturbing comments about the ipilimumab treatment we hoped was coming. "How will we know whether it's been working?" he asked. "You have no tumor, so we can't measure shrinkage. We have no way of monitoring success." Gordon was nonplussed and did not reply. Alone in the car, driving home, however, he thought about what he should have said: "There was no such gauge for the benefits of radiation either. I didn't have a tumor that shrank. But you can measure survival—that is also meaningful." When Gordon told me what he heard, I was distressed. If more people in the agency felt the same way, could that derail Gordon's participation in the compassionate care program?

Effective adjuvant therapy for melanoma was in its infancy. Since other malignancies such as breast cancer had yielded to this approach, we had every reason to believe it could also work with melanoma—if the right drugs were found. Ipilimumab was an approved therapy, and we had some evidence it could prevent recurrence in individuals whose tumors had been removed surgically. Understandably, the radiologist would be more comfortable if we could point to a string of clinical trials demonstrating success. But if Gordon delayed until that happened, he might miss a potentially life-saving drug. He might get sicker; the tumors might return. And while he might have better information, he ran the risk of making it harder to achieve a cure. Waiting for more data was a luxury he couldn't afford. I was surprised the radiologist had so little appreciation for Gordon's predicament.

On August 21, Gordon drove to Lions Gate Hospital and reported to the chemo department for dacarbazine. He walked to the infusion room where he joined about a dozen people being treated for various cancers. He signed in and was told to pick a bed or reclining chair. Gordon lay down and waited. A few minutes later, a nurse came by and hooked him up to a bag containing a pale yellow liquid. After the bag was emptied, she detached him from the machine and Gordon returned home. He was prescribed a handful of medications to ameliorate the side effects of the therapy: Neupogen and Neulasta to boost the supply of white blood cells, which the chemotherapy would reduce, as well as Kytril, Maxeran, and Decadron to prevent nausea. A week later Bristol-Myers Squibb called: Gordon was approved for ipilimumab! He was going to receive it through the company's Access to Hope Program, which provided a variety of services to patients. A welcome package with more information was in the mail and should arrive shortly. I still didn't understand why Gordon was required to have the chemo. Was he supposed to pay his dues in order to be considered eligible for a true remedy? In any case, he'd satisfied the rules and was able to proceed. He couldn't have ipilimumab right away though; four weeks needed to elapse between the infusion of chemotherapy and the injection of ipilimumab. Once this "wash-out" period was over, Gordon could start a course of the new drug. He would get a total of four infusions, at three-week intervals. We had been thinking about this day since March. I could hardly believe it was happening. I felt a fanfare should be played.

We had another reason to celebrate: September 3 was Tom and Leanna's first wedding anniversary. To mark this auspicious occasion, we spent a few days with them and with Pat and Talia, in Ucluelet, a small village on the west coast of Vancouver Island. We weren't in the mood for any big adventures, but we kayaked in the harbor, where we admired a black bear and her cub foraging along the shore. We could hear the stones clattering as Momma Bear overturned them looking for the shellfish underneath. The familiar pleasures of the west coast were there, but with melancholy notes, mostly due to the effects of Tom's concussion. Gordon wrote:

> *The six of us are "camping" at the Water's Edge Resort. Tom instigated this trip. He wanted to go to Cow Bay—by water taxi—but I don't think he'll be able to—nor does he. This concussion still drags on— ten weeks now—and there is talk of progress, but no real measures. It seems hard for him to integrate the different elements of experience into a stable world model. Walking fatigues him; he walks slowly. Car trips are a problem—being in a rapidly moving vehicle. Sensory overload must be avoided. Background music to a dinner conversation must be kept low—very low. His intelligence seems unimpaired—looking over Talia's shoulder while she played Funbridge, he had an impressive grasp of the problem of how to make the contract, the order in which to play the suits, finesses necessary to improve the odds of winning. He is as lively as usual, except when he's tired. And his enthusiasm for doing things is there, although he must restrain himself severely—he swam yesterday at Long Beach, and made cinnamon buns last night, bracketing our riotous crab dinner (not really riotous, but it seemed that way—six crabs, two pots, three crab crackers, six people).*

On September 18, Gordon made his way over to Lions Gate Hospital again. By now he knew the drill. Show up at the chemo department, sign in, find a recliner, wait for the nurses, and allow himself to be infused. He was given a bag of saline solution, then the ipilimumab, and then more saline to make sure that every last drop of the expensive prescription was flushed out of the tube and into his vein. Ipilimumab might overstimulate Gordon's immune system and cause gastrointestinal upset, itchiness, or skin inflammation. But not everyone experienced these symptoms. Some people had remarkably little in the way of side effects so Gordon wasn't given any pills to off-set the effects of the immunotherapy, only told to report bothersome symptoms. Afterward he felt well enough to go up to the lake for ten days—the last gasp of summer.

> *September 23, Sunday, Sheridan Lake. Warm caressing sun. The lake unruffled. Gordon was tired but not too bad—said he felt his insides rumbling—digestive upsets are a known side effect. Supposedly more symptoms will come after the third dose. He's been coughing thinks it's an effect of the radiation.*
>
> *September 26. Gordon's seroma has disappeared just like that— gone. Was it the effect of chopping wood? Canoeing? Using the chainsaw?*
>
> *A cougar was sighted at Edall Bay—made our walk in the woods a little—well, it had a "frisson" to it.*
>
> *I told Gordon, "I find it hard to believe you're over the melanoma." He said, "Why not? Your parents escaped from the Nazis, another grave threat."*

My parents were proof you could pull back from the precipice. The danger they faced and the one in front of Gordon were worlds' apart, but I often drew inspiration from their story, from my father's persistence and his accurate assessment of the situation. As soon as German troops marched into Vienna, he started thinking about how to leave. Some of his friends were convinced their problems would blow over, but my father was not so sanguine. (Like me, he had a tendency to imagine the worst possible outcome!) He escaped to Shanghai, where he and my mother survived World War II. With determination and some luck, you could overcome serious hazards; I had to remember that.

We snugged up the cabin for winter and drove home. Gordon's persistent cough was troubling me. I wrote: *I'm scared, worried that it's cancer.* Was the melanoma in Gordon's lungs? Since I had not been through anything like this, it was always hard to tell when I was seeing an indicator of trouble or a passing and inconsequential phenomenon.

October 4. Gordon thinks the symptoms are "consistent with the physical damage from radiation." I gloom around. He says I shouldn't be on a death watch, says he feels like the woman in Zorba the Greek. Gordon says I am a case.

October 19, Natural Bridges State Park, Santa Cruz, California. A kaleidoscope of orange flecks high up in the eucalyptus trees transfixed us. They were monarch butterflies that had migrated from valleys west of the Rocky Mountains to spend the winter down south. When the butterflies rested, they folded their wings up and over themselves—exposing the dull brown undersides which afforded excellent camouflage. You couldn't see them while they were on their perches, but if a gust of wind or a bird disturbed them, they fluttered away and bright orange shards burst out between the trees. For an hour or so, we watched, charmed by the display, and then drove on. We were holidaying for ten days in California, before going to Gordon's conference. In Monterey, we tried to pay homage to John Steinbeck, whose famous book *Cannery Row* begins, "Cannery Row is a poem, a stink, a grating noise, a quality of light, a tone, a habit, a nostalgia." The street is still there but the last cannery closed in 1973, and there is no stink or poem left. The original residents—Steinbeck's "whores, pimps, gamblers, and sons of bitches"—would be astonished no doubt by the swank restaurants and hotels that now occupy their strip of waterfront on the harbor. More to our taste was Point Lobos Park, south of Monterey. We walked along the roiling ocean and I took many pictures of ochre-colored sandstone, which the sea had molded into rounded, sensuous shapes.

From there, we drove north to San Francisco, where we stayed in a bed and breakfast. We visited the old hippy neighborhood of Haight-Ashbury, rode the cable cars, walked through Chinatown, browsed in the famous City Lights Bookstore, explored the Beat Museum with its Jack Kerouac and Allen Ginsberg memorabilia, and took a Segway tour of Golden Gate Park. We ambled about quite happily. On the last weekend of our trip, we crossed the Golden Gate Bridge to San Rafael, the location of Gordon's conference. The two hundred or so attendees and dozens of presenters came from all over the world to participate in discussions about "The Nature of the Self," but the style of the event was very Californian. A cross-section of seekers had come—white-robed Sufis, orange-robed Buddhists, gurus and would-be gurus, psychologists and therapists in various traditions, a few academics. Cool rationalists like Gordon were in short supply, but he did meet a PhD student in neurology whose work on how we construct our body images intrigued him. Did Gordon make converts to his way of thinking? Probably not. But he had some good conversations and made a few useful contacts. All in all, he thought it worthwhile.

We flew home to sluicing rain and Gordon's next (and third) infusion of ipilimumab. Again he experienced minimal side effects. Instead of being a cause of satisfaction, this was beginning to concern me. I was vividly aware of research showing that patients who experienced significant adverse events were less likely to relapse.[2] To determine whether the ipilimumab was working, we could not monitor shrinking tumors as Gordon's radiologist had so emphatically emphasized. So, though normally one would not welcome digestive upsets or rashes, they would at least indicate Gordon was on the right track. All we could do was wait for new CT scans and see whether he was one of the lucky ones—one of the "responders." As Dr. Wang observed, "After successful treatment and passing through the 'mad rush' phase, many patients initially feel a sense of relief. Soon, however, they develop new questions and concerns."[3]

Dr. Wang had dubbed this second part of the melanoma experience the "marathon." To think of the future stretching out this way—to be long enough to encompass a marathon rather than just a sprint—was agreeable. Less congenial was the idea that this future was going to contain plenty of opportunity for trepidation.

7

THE ICONOCLAST: A VISIT WITH JAMES ALLISON

"**W**hat does our fearless leader's schedule look like today?" the young man asked. The receptionist smiled and said, "Well, he has one interview this morning [that was me], and then a meeting at two and another at three. How much time do you need?" The young man said, "About half an hour." The receptionist shook her head, "Fifteen minutes would be easier." Shrugging his shoulders and grinning, he replied, "Okay, I'll take what I can get." The fearless leader was Dr. James Allison, the man whose revolutionary ideas led to the development of ipilimumab, the immunotherapy upon which Gordon and I had pinned our hopes.

I had come to Houston, Texas, to meet Allison, the chair of the immunology department at the MD Anderson Cancer Center. I felt he was just as much a part of our story as the local doctors who were helping Gordon to recover. Without Allison's inquisitiveness, Gordon's prospects would be dim indeed. I wanted to know what he was like and how he engineered a paradigm shift that was so important to us. Why was he able to see alternatives when others could not? And equally significant, how was he able to persuade people to adopt a new way of thinking?

The idea of using the immune system to cure cancer had a long and somewhat troubled history. The story of what happened to Dr. Steven Rosenberg was often held up as a cautionary tale. He appeared on the cover of *Newsweek* in December 1985 as part of a report about a promising immune system product called interleukin-2. (This was the drug

Kathy took back in 2005.) Hopes ran high that finally a solution for melanoma was at hand: "The experimental therapy unleashes the killing action of the body's white blood cells against tumors; according to NCI director Dr.Vincent T. DeVita Jr., it represents 'the most interesting and exciting biological therapy we've seen so far.'"[1] But excitement gave way to disappointment: only a few people were helped, after all. This pattern seemed to repeat itself over and over again. Immunotherapies developed a reputation for overpromising and underdelivering. But Allison revived their fortunes by taking a contrarian approach. While the majority of investigators asked what turned the immune system on, Allison also inquired into what made it go off. Transforming the question like that made a surprising and profound difference.

While I was thumbing through a magazine, the receptionist gestured to me: I could go in. Allison is much in demand these days. The recipient of a fistful of awards and prizes, he lectures all over the world about his research. I felt quite fortunate that I was able to talk to him. A rumpled, bearded man of sixty-seven, he spoke quietly in a gravelly drawl, a voice that you could easily imagine hearing out on the range somewhere. The day I met him, he was casually dressed in a charcoal sweater and pants. As we talked at a round meeting table strewn with papers, I heard the continual "ping" of the computer on his desk nearby alerting him to incoming e-mail messages.

I knew that Allison had deep roots in Texas, so I started by asking about them. He said he was born in Alice, a small oil town about a hundred miles from the Mexican border. Cactus and mesquite dot the surrounding featureless scrubland on a coastal plain called the Rio Grande Valley. "Everything that's there sticks you, bites you, or stings you," Allison recalled. His family was Scotch-Irish and started ranching in the Lone Star State before the Civil War. "My nephew does a lot of rodeoing, a lot of calf roping. One of his daughters got a barrel riding fellowship to the University of Wyoming. I didn't know there was such a thing," he said, laughing. Allison keeps photographs on his desk, and he showed me a picture of his wife, Dr. Padmanee Sharma, an oncologist, and his son, Robert, an architect in New York.

Cancer scarred Allison's family deeply. When he was eleven years old, his mom developed lymphoma; he was at her bedside when she died. Later, an uncle passed away due to lung cancer. Allison said, "He was a rancher who was in the sun a lot. But he also smoked. He could roll a cigarette while he was on a horse." Another uncle developed melanoma, but refused to be treated after having seen the toll that radiation and chemotherapy took on his siblings. He died too. In 2006, one of Allison's two brothers succumbed to prostate cancer, the same year that he himself was successfully treated for that disease.

Allison's early experiences probably had an influence, he told me, "but it's not that I said, 'I'm going to cure cancer.'" He had a broad curiosity about the world around him; science intrigued him from an early age: "I was fascinated by solving things, understanding things." This made him something of an outsider. "It was Texas," he pointed out. "It was not noted for intellectual pursuits. Wednesdays and Sundays you go to church. Fridays you go to the football game." In high school, Allison recounted, "I was on the verge of boredom most of the time." But he did have a couple of inspired teachers. Stan Brooks, a counselor, got him into summer programs for creative students at the University of Texas in Austin, and his math teacher, Ernestine Glossbrenner, made algebra come alive for him. "She and I were friends for a long time," Allison said. But his biology class was a wasteland. Allison caused an uproar when he discovered it would not include any mention of evolution. "You quoted Newton when you were teaching physics, so how can you teach biology without a unifying principle?" he asked his teacher. He refused to fritter his days away on such a curriculum. A compromise was reached when Brooks suggested he take a correspondence course, which did include the study of evolution.

After graduating from high school at sixteen, Allison entered the University of Texas at Austin, a city he had grown to appreciate during his summers there. "I was born in Alice," he said, "but I grew up in Austin." Allison enrolled in a premed program, partly because his father, who was a doctor, was hoping he would follow in his footsteps. Soon Allison realized that temperamentally, he was not suited to be a physician. "You have to be right. You don't have a lot of room to mess around." He shifted over to science. "It's more fun, because you can be wrong. You can be wrong a lot. You *are* wrong a lot," he said with a smile. In his senior year, Allison got a taste for the allure of immunotherapy during an experiment he did with mice that he had cured of leukemia. On a whim, he decided to see whether they could be reinfected. The mice proved resistant, and he realized they had acquired an immune response. "I was just screwing around," he said, "but that impressed me." Allison got his BSc in microbiology and stayed on at the university to do a PhD in biochemistry.

In 1974, Allison took up a postdoc fellowship in La Jolla, California, at the Scripps lab, which had a reputation for being one of the "hottest" places in the country for immunology. But Allison was disgruntled:

> I didn't like the lab I was in in La Jolla, it was old style. Old style, meaning pyramid. They would hire two people, put them on close to the same project. Whoever was the most aggressive would win. It was okay. I could hold my own. But I didn't like it. I wanted to do something different. I realized they would have me doing biochemistry the whole time I was there. I wanted to figure out what was going on. I wanted to understand. Having a technique and having your life dominated by a technique was not my idea of what I wanted to do. I wanted to define issues that fascinated me and work on those, whatever it takes.

Allison's outlet while in La Jolla was music. He played the harmonica and he remembered, "I met these guys on the beach in San Diego and started playing with them. Every Tuesday and most Fridays, we played at this bar in Encinitas called the Stingree." The "guys" were Clay Blaker and the Texas Honky Tonk Band (who are still going strong). The association led to a remarkable evening. Willie Nelson's album *Red-Headed Stranger* had just gone platinum, so Columbia Records held a party for him in San Diego. Allison snuck into the festivities and struck up a conversation with Nelson. When the singer mentioned that he was looking for somewhere to play the next night, Allison invited him to talent night at his usual hang-out, the Stingree. There, Allison played a little harmonica as Nelson was opening with "Blue Eyes Crying in the Rain." It was quite a moment. Later, when Blaker decided to go on a Texas tour in an area known as "The German Dance Circuit" between San Antonio and Austin, he invited Allison to join him. Allison turned him down, although he still plays gigs with two groups of music-loving scientists, the Checkmates and the Checkpoints. (You can catch the latter band at the American Society of Clinical Oncology conferences, where they often provide the entertainment.)

Allison declined to go to Texas for music, but nonetheless went back in 1977. MD Anderson offered him a faculty position at a small research center in Smithville. The job attracted Allison because the lab was just forty miles southeast of Austin, Allison's favourite city. In Smithville, Allison could pursue some of the scientific questions that deeply interested him.

He also picked up the cudgel for a cause close to his heart—the importance of good science education. His fight began with a call from his former math teacher, Glossbrenner. In 1976, she ran for public office and was elected as a Democrat to the Texas House of Representatives. She phoned Allison because of a bill that Mike Martin, a freshman Republican legislator, introduced during the 1981 session. It would require that public schools give equal time to the study of creationism and the theory of evolution. Glossbrenner said, "Jim, you've got to come down here and help. If there's nobody to oppose this, the bill will have to go up to the floor." So Allison, who was passionate about science and never shy about speaking his mind, rode to the rescue. He recalled telling Martin:

> It's not just accounting for the past. It's something you can use. I can use the thoughts of selection in my work, to find out how bacteria become resistant to antibiotics. I can use the Darwinian ideas about evolution to explain how a cancer cell evolves, escapes the immune system. We can use the lessons of biology to help us make drugs, to get better crops. Can your creation science do that? The TV cameras were there and I got up and said, "I'll challenge this man to tell me anything that creation science can be used for in the real world."

The bill was sent to a committee for further study and never came to a vote. Martin was later named one of the "Ten Worst Legislators" in the July 1981 *Texas Monthly*.[2]

Allison was fascinated by T cells. They are lymphocytes, white blood cells that are produced in the bone marrow and mature in the thymus, from which they get their name. The thymus is a small organ located between the lungs. T cells destroy other cells that are dangerous because they harbor pathogens or are defective in some way. They bind to bad cells, poke holes in their membranes, and inject them with an arsenal of lethal enzymes. The average person has about one billion T cells—one of several kinds of white blood cells our bodies use to rid us of disease.

We, their hosts, mostly tolerate this chemical warfare within. "They don't kill you. *Why* don't they kill you?" Allison asked me with a gleam in his eye, clearly still intrigued by the phenomenon. When Allison arrived in Smithville, T cells were the source of many mysteries. What activated them? How did they distinguish unhealthy tissues from normal ones? Why did they kill viruses so efficiently, but for the most part leave cancer cells alone? In 1982, Allison made a breakthrough that helped to answer some of these questions—the discovery of T cell antigen receptors. They are sensor molecules on the surface of T cells that let them identify diseased cells. A cell infected by a microbe displays an antigen on its surface, part of the interloper that spells trouble. Each T cell has a set of approximately twenty thousand identical receptors that allow it to recognize a specific antigen. If a T cell patrolling the body meets that complementary antigen, one of its receptors will bind with it. (Antigen and receptor fit together rather like a hand in a glove.) Discovering these receptors was a major step forward. In fact, it was so important it was known as the Holy Grail of immunology. But as is so often the case in science, the finding led to more questions. Allison explained, "People began to realize that if you try to stimulate a naïve T cell just by hitting the T cell antigen receptor, it's not enough, it won't go. It's like the ignition of a car." If you turn the switch, the engine goes on, but the car still won't move. Before T cells could destroy faulty cells, something else besides an antigen receptor was involved. What was it?

After Allison published his discovery about T cell receptors, the University of California at Berkeley offered him a job as chairman of the department of immunology. He left Texas in 1984, and in his lab in California he began searching for a "co-stimulatory molecule" that would spur T cells into action. Allison turned his attention to CD28, another protein on the surface of T cells. He decided from what he had seen of other scientists' research about CD28 that "it smelled right." His instinct was bang-on. After investigating further, Alison found that CD28 provided "an essential second signal." Activating it was "like hitting the gas pedal." CD28 could give a T cell several positive messages, including the signal to divide after it recognized a diseased cell. This created a whole cohort of T cells able to find and destroy cells with the same defect. When the troupe had done its work, most of its members died, but a few remained on stand-by as memory cells, should the sickness return.

Meanwhile, the scientific community had become interested in another protein sometimes found on T cells—CTLA-4. Discovered in 1987,[3] it resembled CD28, and many people, including Allison, thought it was potentially another booster. However, on closer inspection, he found that CTLA-4 seemed to inhibit T cell division—the opposite of what you'd expect if the molecule was an accelerant. While other scientists continued to look for evidence that it was a stimulatory molecule, Allison was struck by the possibility that CTLA-4 might be a brake on the immune system. Scientists had not thought much about inhibition systems, but it stood to reason that if there were Go signals, there would also be Stop signals. Maybe CTLA-4 was the answer to the long-standing riddle about why cancers so often evaded the immune system. By then, investigators knew that cancer cells, like viruses and bacteria, had antigens that could trigger an immune response.[4] Researchers also realized that T cells occasionally destroyed malignant cells.[5] However, even when they did this, the T cells seemed incapable of finishing the job and ridding the body of cancer. Allison entertained the radical hypothesis that CTLA-4 was crippling the T cells' offensive. What would happen if he took off the restraint?

In 1995, Max Krummel, now a professor in the department of pathology at the University of California, San Francisco, was one of Allison's PhD students at Berkeley. He told me in a phone conversation that Allison was a "sink or swim mentor." Krummel said, "I swam pretty hard." Under Allison's supervision, Krummel created an antibody to CTLA-4 as part of his thesis project. Early experiments in vitro—with cells in petri dishes—established that by applying the antibody you could block CTLA-4 and cause T cells to proliferate. By withholding it, you could reverse the effect—activate the CTLA-4 and inhibit the division of T cells. Of course, Allison wanted to see what would happen in vivo—in live animals. Allison gave Dana Leach, one of his research fellows, who was also a veterinarian, the task of implanting mice with colon cancer. Then he asked him to treat some of them with the antibody to CTLA-4. If the brake on the immune system was lifted, would this be enough to destroy the tumors? And equally important, would the mice survive this manipulation? Or would they suffer from a devastating autoimmune disorder?

In November 1995, Leach showed Allison the results of the experiment. In the untreated mice, the tumors grew so large, the mice had to be euthanized. But in the treated mice, the results were astonishing. The T cells managed to neutralize the tumors with remarkable efficiency. They were almost all gone. Allison said, "I was surprised and delighted. But I'm a cynic and a skeptic. I wondered if I could disprove the results." Leach was going away for his Christmas vacation, but Allison didn't want to wait. He asked Leach to set up the experiment again (and blind it) so that he could monitor it himself over the holidays. For a second time, the mice were given an antibody to interfere with the action of CTLA-4. "When I was measuring the tumors, I didn't know which box was which," Allison told me. Initially, the results were disheartening. All the mice were the same. Their cancers grew and more of them were developing. Allison became despondent. "I skipped a measurement or two because I didn't want to get more depressed," he said. When he finally came back to the lab, he got a delayed Christmas present. He could see that in one group of mice, the tumor growth was starting to slow down. Then the cancers began shrinking and eventually went away altogether. At six weeks, when the experiment was unblinded, he realized that most of the treated mice were fine—90 percent of their tumors were gone. None of the untreated mice survived.

Allison repeated the experiment in different ways, using different strains of mice and different kinds of tumors—kidney cancer, leukemia, breast cancer, melanoma. He also did an experiment reminiscent of the one he had done as an undergraduate. When five mice that had never received the antibody to CTLA-4 were injected with colon cancer cells, they developed lethal tumors in a couple of weeks. On the other hand, when five mice that had been successfully treated with the antibody were reinjected with malignant cells, three of them rejected the tumors and remained healthy. This was evidence, Allison wrote, that the treatment "results in immunologic memory."[6]

Allison emphasized that CTLA-4 was part of the normal functioning of the immune system. As soon as the T cell is activated, it begins to make CTLA-4. "It's hard-wired in the process to stop the immune system," Allison said. It appears on the surface of the T cell a few days after it is switched on and "pushes CD28 out of the way," Allison explained. Another experiment Allison and some other researchers did revealed the consequences of not having any CTLA-4 at all. Mice from which the gene for CTLA-4 was deleted died within three weeks of being born because their T cells couldn't stop proliferating. So, having no CTLA-4 was disastrous. Fortunately, the antibody to it had a half-life of about two weeks. So it only obstructed the CTLA-4 brake temporarily, and, in mice at least, this seemed to prevent autoimmune disease.

Since T cells usually manage to dispatch germ-infected cells without any such intervention, I was curious about what made cancer so different. When I asked Allison about that, he offered a speculation. He said, "This is my idea. A lot of people don't like it. You won't read it in a text book, but I think it explains a lot. It's a question of sequence." T cells are good at killing viruses, he observed. "You can go from one hundred in your body to ten to twenty million in three or four days. Because they are so efficient, that's enough time to deal with the viruses. But with a tumor, you need more time." This made sense to me. A tumor was much larger than a virus; I could see why destroying it might take more than a few days. By temporarily impeding CTLA-4, the antibody gave the T cells an extension—the leeway they needed to kill the tumors.

Once Allison had demonstrated how the CTLA-4 antibody worked in mice, the next step was to try it in humans. Allison began approaching pharmaceutical companies to see if they wanted to take on this project. To his dismay, they kept turning him down. Allison explained, "By then, the prejudice against immunotherapy was so deep." Over the years, it became clear that attempts to destroy cancer by boosting the immune system didn't work very well. Though Allison was proposing something different—blocking a blocker to the immune system—it didn't inspire much confidence either. Allison spoke to about a dozen corporations and made a few false starts with companies that licensed his discovery but did nothing with it. Then a small pharmaceutical company based in New Jersey, Medarex, took the plunge. It created a human version of the antibody that Allison was using on mice. In 1999, the company launched a small phase I experiment, designed to see whether people could tolerate the therapy. If they could, other trials would follow to compare its ability to cure people with that of standard treatments. Fourteen people participated. They were stage IV melanoma patients who had failed to benefit from several different therapies. Their outlook was bleak. After receiving the antibody (eventually called ipilimumab), three of the patients responded, and in two of those three, the tumors disappeared completely.[7]

Allison recalled, "They [the investigators] went 'Wow, this doesn't happen in a safety trial.' Normally, in a safety trial, you just want to be sure you didn't hurt the patients." In July 2003, the National Academy of Sciences published a paper about the experiment. The authors, including Allison, describe a watershed moment in medicine, but their language is restrained: "This clinical trial has indicated a potential role for CTLA-4 blockade in cancer immunotherapy."[8]

Later, said Allison, he met a woman who had responded in this original trial. She is still alive, he told me, and was able to see her children grow up, establish themselves, and start families of their own. "I'm not a clinician, I don't get to see that very often," he remarked, a little wistfully, I thought. Behind the dry statistics about response rates there are individuals with heartrending histories. Most of the patients in the trial did not get a positive result. They were probably crushed to hear that even this last-ditch attempt with an unproven therapy had not worked. Only a select lucky two must have been elated when they found out the cancer was in retreat and they could get on with their lives.

In 2004, Allison moved again, to the Sloan Kettering Cancer Center in New York to become chair of the immunology program there. He took the job because he wanted to be close to some of the clinicians who were conducting the major trials—to lend his advice and help shepherd the drug home. Like a mom who was determined that her talented (but shy) offspring get the credit they deserved, Allison advocated tirelessly on behalf of his therapy:

> Additionally, researchers in basic immunology should not be reluctant to assertively engage with clinicians and companies, an endeavor that goes far beyond simply "outlicensing" a patent and then retreating to the sidelines. Jim Allison, who has no medical degree, was the paragon of this model as the anti-CTLA-4 "promotor in chief," he engaged, badgered, charmed and cajoled whomever was in a position to move the therapy forward.[9]

By January 2005, Medarex attracted a much larger collaborator, Bristol-Myers Squibb, and together, the two companies conducted more trials.

Even though the first safety trial was successful, the path ahead was rocky. On March 16, 2006, a small safety trial in England of another immunotherapy went spectacularly wrong, a major setback for the field. The medicine was a CD28 super-agonist—a stimulatory antibody designed to give CD28 an immense boost. Only six human volunteers participated in the trial; each was given a dose five hundred times smaller than the one observed to be safe in earlier animal experiments. But within minutes of receiving the medication, the previously healthy men "moaned in uncontrollable pain, vomited and struggled for breath."[10] All suffered multiple organ failure and were transferred to an intensive care unit. Two were placed on ventilators. They survived but their experience led to a lot of soul searching among researchers and to new guidelines concerning the conduct of clinical trials.[11] The result was certainly a sobering reminder that the immune system is a powerful instrument and that you need to be careful when you manipulate it.

In December 2007, another disaster: a Medarex phase II trial of ipilimumab with 155 melanoma patients was deemed a failure. It hadn't reached its primary goal of shrinking the tumors of at least 10 percent of the patients.[12] Then on April 2, 2008, Pfizer announced it was shutting down a phase III trial of a drug called tremelimumab, which like ipilimumab was a CTLA-4 blocker.[13] According to Pfizer, the trial involving another 655 people with melanoma showed the drug was no better than standard chemotherapy. "That alarmed us," said Allison. But he believed the problems were not so much with the drugs as with the way in which they were evaluated. For a chemotherapy drug, three months was typically the decisive moment. If it had not worked by then, continuing was futile. The medicine would fail at six months too. But immunotherapy appeared to be quite different. Evidence started trickling in that some people whose tumors were still growing at three months experienced remissions later on. Allison explained:

> What you do is a CAT scan or something like that. You measure the entire body load of cancer at base line. You start giving the drug. Then you look again, typically at three months, and measure again. It can only be called an objective response, if there is greater than 51 percent shrinkage. In addition, no tumor can have gotten bigger and you can't have any new tumors. A couple of randomized trials were set up early on. Progression-free survival was the end point. As soon as a patient's tumor starts growing, it's over. So they're off the trial because there's progressive disease, no response. And a month later, the tumors would disappear. That was missed sometimes.
>
> In the early trials, people were referred to big cancer centers. As soon as they'd progressed, they'd be told, "We're sorry it didn't work,

go back to your community doctor." They would go on to chemo or something. No chemo drugs ever worked [for melanoma] but people would do that anyway. Sometimes patients would do very well. I remember hearing these stories—that chemo works better after CTLA-4. Well, the chemo might not have had anything to do with it.

People were seeing patients who'd respond late—at six months even. Several guys that I know starting telling BMS, "I have patients, they failed the trial, but they are still coming back two years later." Reports started coming in. People like Jedd [Dr. Jedd Wolchok] and Steve [Dr. Stephen Hodi] told BMS what was happening. They changed the endpoint on their big trial from progression-free survival to overall survival. The only criterion was that you were alive. You could have tumors all over, but if you were alive, you were in. The drug worked but the trial design was wrong.

The big trial to which Allison referred opened in September 2004. A phase III study, it enrolled a total of 675 patients at 125 centers in thirteen countries. The participants, who all had stage IV melanoma, were put on one of three regimes—ipilimumab, ipilimumab plus a vaccine, or a vaccine alone. In the early 1990s scientists began to use their knowledge of cancer antigens to create vaccines that could trigger an immune response and eliminate malignancies.[14] Unlike the vaccines that are most familiar to us, they did not prevent disease, but were given after its onset to prod the immune system into action. On paper, the approach sounded good; in practice, success rates were frustratingly low, not much better than chemotherapy. Still, the vaccine was used as a point of comparison.

When the trial started, its aim was to discover which of these three approaches was best able to shrink tumors. But in January 2009, while the trial was still blinded, Bristol-Myers Squibb took the unusual step of asking the U.S. Food and Drug Administration (FDA) to approve a new way of measuring success—survival.[15] This was a little like moving the goal posts after the game had started. However, the FDA allowed BMS to make the change in view of the evidence about "late" responders. A 2010 report revealed that the patients who received ipilimumab alone lived longest. At the two-year mark, 23.5 percent were alive. Allison recalled that, even more remarkably, most of these patients were still alive four years later. Oncologists call this "a durable response." In less understated language, you might venture to describe it as a "cure." No other drug had achieved anything remotely similar for melanoma.

Allison emphasized the differences between the therapy he had helped to devise and earlier ones: "My work says you're treating the immune system first of all, not the cancer. That is a very important thing. I had to remind the oncologists, 'Don't treat this like a cancer drug. It's not a cancer drug at all.'" Allison also stressed that the ipilimumab wasn't intended to boost the immune system. "We're doing the opposite. We're trying to keep it from turning itself *off*—to keep the immune system going." Earlier immunotherapies tried to stimulate the immune system, but unless you release the brake first, the push has little effect.

The T cells still had to recognize the cancer and destroy it—a significant advantage. With older therapies, you always had to worry about the cancer developing ways of evading them. Allison said, "Since the war on cancer started more than forty years ago, we've learned so much about tumor cells, about their growth and about what causes cancer at the molecular basis. It's beautiful, amazing work, much of which has been made possible by genome sequencing and the identification of driver mutations." Despite this, tumors find a way around anticancer drugs. They *evolve*. But now, Allison said, "If you keep the immune system going, and there are new mutations, it will see them too. The escape mechanisms don't matter." You have to remember that we have millions of T cells—each with their own unique set of antigen receptors. En masse, they can recognize pretty much anything thrown at them.

Because ipilimumab lets the immune system do the heavy lifting, it manages the astonishing feat of being both very general in its application and highly specific. Allison said that in addition to benefitting patients with melanoma, ipilimumab can help those with kidney, prostate, and bladder cancer. Anecdotal reports point to its efficacy with ovarian and pancreatic cancer, as well as glioblastoma. At the same time, Allison said, "it's highly individualized. It may be specific to one person's melanoma. You don't have to work at making it individualized. Your immune system does that."

Although the new immunotherapy is quite different from old treatments, it can work synergistically with them. When radiation or drugs kill tumor cells, the dying cells release antigens, creating an ideal situation for T cells to recognize them and to become primed. Furthermore, the T cells give you memory. After they destroy a cancer, Allison explained, "a lot of them die, but some of them go into this dormant state and they slowly renew themselves and you've got them for the rest of your life." Your body remembers that cancer, and should the mutation appear again, it's prepared and can mount an assault much more rapidly than it did at first.

Allison steered a course to a new world of immunotherapy. No longer do inventors have to struggle to get these therapies accepted. "They are just sailing into the clinic," said Allison. The "off switches" are called checkpoints, and the novel pharmaceuticals are called checkpoint blockades. (Allison's band, the Checkpoints, also takes its name from these therapies.)

Allison and I talked for a couple of hours, and then I had to go. Graciously, he walked with me to the elevator and out to the parking lot. We shook hands while standing in the pale winter sunlight and I thanked Allison for his time. When I was riding in a taxi through north Houston, to George Bush International Airport, passing the endless industrial parks, the parking lots, the sprawling one-story factories and commercial buildings, I was thinking about Allison. I thought that what I really should have thanked him for was his curiosity, his determination, his willingness to challenge conventional thinking. Without that, where would Gordon and so many other melanoma patients be?

8

A CLOUD OF UNCERTAINTY

Scanitis, or *scanxiety*, is what some cancer patients call it—the particular misgivings they feel before having a test and afterward, while waiting for the report. I wasn't the one having the scans, but I certainly experienced the anxiety.

> *April 11. Gordon had his CT yesterday. I am scared of the results— no particular reason—just scared!*

On its website, the Mayo Clinic provides some ideas about how to cope with this understandable fear. It suggests keeping busy, meditating, and getting exercise. Further, it advises educating yourself about the signs and symptoms of recurrence for your cancer to have a better sense of what's normal and what's not.[1] When I searched Google for *anxiety cancer scans*, I found 1.4 million results on the topic generally as well as 43,000 scholarly articles. Some of those recommended reducing the number of surveillance scans to spare patients stress.[2] But it was hard to see how this could be safely done with a cancer as dangerous as melanoma.

After several days of anticipatory dread (mostly mine) Gordon and I took our usual places in the examination room at Lions Gate Hospital. He and I sat on two chairs side by side next to the wall, and Dr. Smiljanic sat on the hospital bed. Without much ado, Dr. Smiljanic gave us the news: the recent CT scan showed two worrisome centimeter-sized spots. Neither was in an area you would normally expect to find metastasizing melanoma. The lungs, liver, bones, axilla were all clear, but Gordon had one spot in his buttock and another, more indistinct, on the wall of his colon—on the outside, near his liver. The report described both as "suspicious" for metastasis.

"Can you feel anything?" Dr. Smiljanic asked.

Gordon wriggled on his chair a bit and shook his head. "They are looking very hard," Dr. Smiljanic commented.

So we were back in the thick of things, back to distressing lumps of unknown provenance. The CT scan sparked a flurry of further investigations. And then, at the end of the month, on a beautiful cloudless day, Dr. Smiljanic gave us the verdict: an ultrasound and biopsy confirmed a cancer in Gordon's buttock, already a little larger than it was on the CT scan, 1.4 cm in diameter. Dr. Smiljanic said he would order a PET scan to see if there were more tumors.

I was numb, not thinking very clearly.

"We were . . . planning a trip . . ." I said haltingly. We'd made arrangements to visit friends in Ottawa and relatives of Gordon's in Philadelphia and we were about to leave in a few days.

"How long will you be out of town?" Dr. Smiljanic asked.

"About two weeks."

"That's fine. The scan won't happen right away. If I were you, I'd go. I'll set things up; the timing isn't that critical." Dr. Smiljanic added that he was going to order a reexamination of the malignant tissue. He explained that sometimes when patients have taken ipilimumab, you can see T cells invading the tumors. If a pathology report found evidence of this, it would mean the therapy was starting to work and would be a good outcome. At home, I tried to remind myself of the positives. The lump was small. Gordon couldn't even feel it. Critical organs were unaffected—nothing in the lungs, brain, or liver. Maybe the ipilimumab was doing something after all—gradually stirring an army of languorous T cells to belligerence. Dr. Smiljanic had held out hope this might be the case. Still it was hard to see the change as anything but a setback since the melanoma had spread beyond Gordon's lymph nodes and he was now stage IV. I didn't bother to look at the statistics; I knew they wouldn't be cheering. Gordon, usually so steady, was also shaken:

> I feel a bit as though I'd been pole-axed. The thing in my right buttock turned out to be melanoma. I had thought perhaps that battle had been fought and won. But the enemy still lurks.

Even Dr. Smiljanic, who had given us some reason to hope, showed his uneasiness in his records:

> I am very concerned about the small abdominal mass mentioned near the liver. If indeed the disease is not localized to the gluteal lesion then we will need to consider further systemic therapy for Gordon, although I am not sure what exactly as he has just finished ipilimumab in November with thus far very little effect.[3]

Sitting at the gate, waiting for take-off at the Vancouver airport, I spread my diary over my knees. While an anonymous female voice announced final boarding calls, I wrote:

> *May 2. Feel awful. The cancer is full of nasty surprises. I am oppressed by the thought that we should not be on this trip. We should be at home dealing with the issue.*

We went to Ottawa first, where we stayed with friends we had known since university days. We took long walks together along the Ottawa River and recalled the past. Even though I was still worrying about Gordon's upcoming PET scan, at least I wasn't stewing all the time. The four of us laughed, remembering a New Year's Eve party in an attic with rather too much Zinfandel imbibed and a precipitous descent down a steep staircase in the wee hours of the morning. While having dinner together in a Vietnamese restaurant, we caught up on events, happy and not so happy. The Mayo Clinic had missed out on a piece of good advice: seek the company of like-minded souls.

On May 4, we flew to Philadelphia to see Gordon's favorite cousin, Mary, and her husband—both lively people. Their stimulating influence helped to push back the dark anxiety, but did not banish it entirely. Mary lives in an old, quiet house with thick stone walls. On our first night there, Gordon and I fell asleep readily under a green coverlet in a small upstairs room. I had not been thinking much about melanoma before going to bed, but soon a wave of fear rose out of the shoals of my unconscious and tossed me awake. *What if Dr. Smiljanic is wrong and this is critical?* I stared at the dusky walls; I didn't know how to answer the question. Without disturbing Gordon, I nestled closer to him. For a while, I listened to his regular breathing and watched his peaceful form. My unruly ragged terror abated.

The next night, as Gordon and I were talking in bed, in a desultory fashion, I returned to our bête noire. I said, "Sometimes I consider your story and pretend I am hearing it told about somebody else, someone I know only slightly. I'm trying to be objective, to take the personal bias out of my assessment—to be as realistic as possible. Of course, I'm sympathetic to this imaginary patient but I don't rate his chances very high."

"You have a point," Gordon paused. "But don't blight the time we have together, when I feel happy and strong, when you have me, by anticipating *not* having me."

"I feel envious of other people."

"Envy is a dark emotion—a worm. Envy is heavy. Just chuck it."

Spiritual boot camp! I exclaimed in my diary.

Mary offered to take us sightseeing to New York, only a couple of hours away from Philadelphia. We thought a day trip might be fun, so we went. We wandered along Manhattan's High Line, a 1.5-mile linear park built on an old elevated railroad spur. Flowers poke through the unused track and trees are planted there, in places so densely they form thickets twenty-five feet above the street. Sculptures, whimsical and serious, dot the way and you can catch views of worn brownstone buildings juxtaposed against sleek modern glass and steel structures. Both tourists and songbirds flock to the High Line, for its quixotic sylvan pleasures. We had lunch in an Italian restaurant and then visited the sobering Ground Zero commemoration of 9/11. I took pictures everywhere, many of reflections—reflections of the city in slicks of water pooling on cobblestone streets and on the glassy sides of skyscrapers. I was content with the photographs and all that we had seen, but still the day was overlaid with sadness.

We kept hoping for an e-mail from Dr. Smiljanic about the reexamination of the tumor. But by May 10, we had no word.

"If it were good news, we would have heard," I said.

"Not necessarily." Gordon thought we often got the future wrong. He liked to point out that we were right "just enough to get by," but that we were more often mistaken than correct. He'd ask me, "Why make yourself miserable with dire predictions?" But I found it hard to be agnostic. I always wanted to come down on one side or the other, to paint a picture of what lay before us, even if I didn't like it. I think it gave me a feeling of control. Maybe it was illusory; nevertheless, I derived some satisfaction from it.

Then Mary offered a second excursion—to visit her daughter, Linda, whom we had never met. Mary had placed her for adoption when she was born but left a letter and an address with her, should she want to reconnect. Many years later, she did. Linda was now married and had a family of her own. She lived near Washington, D.C., only two hours away. "Do you want to go?" Mary asked. Gordon was eager; this was even more exciting than New York! We traveled with Mary south and arrived around noon. For a few hours we did some sightseeing in Washington, explored the National Mall, toured a museum and the Lincoln Memorial where we stared up at the colossal sculpture of Abraham Lincoln. Then we took in the statue of Martin Luther King, not quite as massive as Lincoln's, but equally impressive. We marveled at how different it all was from Ottawa, where there were monuments, too, but not such grand towering ones. In the late afternoon, Linda's husband picked us up and drove us to their home, where Linda and her boys greeted us warmly. We had dinner with them and then in the morning, over breakfast, Linda told us her story, how she and her adoptive father had found Mary in Sag Harbor and how their relationship had gradually deepened over the years. Then Gordon told Linda about his mom, Charlotte. When Mary was thinking about an abortion, Charlotte had suggested she consider adoption. "These things can work out well, you know," she had said. Looking at Linda and her affectionate family, and thinking about his mom's role in that outcome, Gordon's eyes filled with tears. I was glad we had come. Yes, I'd had misgivings about the trip and wondered if we weren't sufficiently vigilant about the cancer. We had taken a risk; melanoma was a tough opponent. But at that moment, it seemed to me that if you let it set the entire agenda, you were conceding too much. After sharing some more stories and a few hugs, we had to go. We had a train to catch. We posed for photographs in the bright sunshine on the front lawn and promised each other a longer visit on another occasion.

A few days later, waiting in the Philly airport for our flight, I was in thrall to melanoma again, occupied with what awaited us at home.

May 16. Nervous. Gordon has his scan tomorrow. What will it reveal?

I told Gordon I was flinching from what lay ahead. "I dread that appointment, when we'll get the results," I said. Gordon maintained stoutly, "It is what it is." Nothing we thought, felt, or did would change the outcome. When we knew more, we might be able to make better or worse decisions—influence our fate. Then we could reflect about it productively. All we could do now was wait.

A soft grey day in Vancouver, mild and undemanding. I was plagued by a sense of loss. I looked at things around our house—the visible emanations of my relationship with Gordon. I gazed at the Kwakiutl mask he gave me one Christmas. It had a lengthy beak that you could snap open and shut by tugging on a string. Long strands of cedar bark flowed down from its neck. During ceremonies in the shortest days of winter, dancers wore masks like this one, transforming themselves into legendary fierce birds capable of eating human beings. The sharp clap of their beaks probably sent shivers down the spines of the watchers, reminding them how vulnerable they were to predatory and bad spirits. I glanced over our sofa at a photograph of the wintry Murtle River. Its slate grey water ran sluggish, mostly iced up. Gordon took the picture during a skiing holiday in Wells Grey Park, about six hours north of Vancouver. We had it blown up and Gordon framed it. And then my eyes fell upon a batik painting filled with peaked-roof houses and small cars, rounded like Volkswagen Beetles. They were sitting over a kind of poem, "little houses/ and big trees/ sunny billboards/ by the sea/ soda cracker city." We bought the batik years ago at a craft fair to celebrate my first sale of a story. I thought about what it would be like to look at these things without Gordon. Would I stay here? I didn't know.

Gordon wrote:

May 19. Where from here? I'm in a cloud of uncertainty until I know what the PET scan shows. Despite all my ideas, I am attached to my life. I want to do more—have Linda and family up to the Lake, live with Claudia some years yet, see Tom recovered from his concussion and launched in his career, hold a grandchild or two, see the back end of Stephen Harper. If I kept on, it could be a long list! Life without caring what happens is no life at all. I can, and do, take delight in the ongoing lives of people I love.

I wrote:

I feel like on Tuesday I will find out whether I will be hanged or not.

9

A HAIRY WEEK SO FAR

May 21, 2013. "The PET scan results are not good," Dr. Charmaine Kim-Sing said, shaking her head. Gordon and I looked at each other. I took a deep breath: *Here it comes.* Sitting in a cramped room with dull beige walls, we watched Dr. Kim-Sing as she read from a piece of paper. "As well as the tumor in the buttock that you already knew about, there are smaller ones in the right chest wall, the left chest wall, and the upper abdomen."

"That's four," I said.

"Wait," she said. "There's more. There's one near the colon and one in the mesentery. Six, altogether."

"What's the mesentery?" I felt I should ask *something*, and this, though not of utmost importance, was the first question that came to mind. I looked at Dr. Kim-Sing intently, and she explained, but nothing sank in. It was as if she were suddenly speaking a foreign language. (Later I looked up *mesentery* and discovered it's the tissue that attaches the intestines to the abdominal wall.)

"What's my prognosis?" Gordon wanted to know.

"The good news here is that the melanoma is not in any of the major organs."

Yeah, but how long can Gordon stave it off? I thought. *I know he feels well so far, but this cancer is so aggressive.*

"If melanoma goes to the brain, you have four to six months, if it goes to the liver or lungs, nine to twelve," Dr. Kim-Sing told us.

"What's next?" Gordon asked.

"At this point, there are too many tumors to treat with radiation. You need a systemic treatment."

"You mean ipilimumab?" I asked.

"Something like that."

"Gordon already had it and it didn't work. Have you seen people who responded to a second round, when they didn't respond to the first?"

Dr. Kim-Sing nodded. "Yes, I have. You just have to hope for the best and prepare for the worst."

I knew she meant to be encouraging, but I thought she was telling Gordon to get his affairs in order, make plans to die, while at the same time counseling him not to be too gloomy, because of a remote chance things could turn around. I preferred another mantra that Gordon was fond of quoting. It described a strategy for winning at bridge: "Assume the contract can be made." This involved imagining what winning would look like and then thinking about the steps necessary to get there. While it didn't guarantee success, at least it directed your intellectual energy toward a positive outcome. The attitude was better than hope. *Hope is too passive,* I thought.

We spent about ten minutes with Dr. Kim-Sing. The upshot was that she couldn't do anything for Gordon. Radiation was Dr. Kim-Sing's specialty, and Dr. Smiljanic had made an appointment with her for Gordon, in case he could be treated by radiation. Now it seemed a systemic treatment, a drug therapy of some kind, was appropriate and that was Dr. Smiljanic's responsibility. We'd have to discuss it with him.

We were pretty quiet as we walked to the car, both of us sunk into ourselves. "How are you today?" the parking attendant asked, as we rolled up to his booth and paid. Gordon didn't say anything. I was still shell-shocked and I thought, *We've just received a death sentence.* We'd had such high expectations about ipilimumab, the most advanced therapy available to us. Health Canada gave it the green light in February 2012, a month before Gordon was diagnosed. We thought it was extraordinary luck that it was available. But now it had failed us. Would it work on a second attempt? And if not? It struck me as pretty unlikely that the older therapies would be effective if ipi wasn't.

As we drove over the Cambie Street viaduct to North Vancouver, I asked Gordon, "What do you think your odds are?"

"Not good." And then he turned to me. "I guess I should have applied for my CPP a little earlier," he said, and laughed. He was talking about our pension. You can get it when you turn sixty, but if you wait until you're sixty-five, the monthly payments are larger. Gordon comes from long-lived stock, so he calculated that this way, he would do better financially. I laughed too.

Gordon e-mailed Sasha to tell him the latest: "I saw Dr. Kim-Sing today and got the report, which I understand you've not yet seen. Unfortunately, it shows 6 spots."

May 22. I was formulating a plan. When I first heard about lambrolizumab, I thought of a lizard, green and scaly with a flashing tail and golden eyes—just the thing for striking a cold, unfeeling enemy such as melanoma. Developed by Merck, lambrolizumab was an immunotherapy like ipilimumab. But it released a different brake on the T cells—PD-1. (For that reason, the drug was sometimes called an anti-PD-1 therapy.) In a preliminary study, lambrolizumab helped 35 percent of patients, whereas its cousin, ipilimumab, achieved responses in fewer people—10 to 20 percent.[1] Although not yet approved in either the United States or Canada, the therapy looked so promising, the U.S. FDA had granted it "breakthrough" status in April 2013 to expedite acceptance.[2]

I knew the U.S. agency would not ratify lambro for another year or two and Health Canada would take even longer. Gordon could not afford to wait. For him, enrolling in a clinical trial looked like the only way to access the drug in a timely fashion. Even though our last attempts to get him into a study had failed, I thought that we might succeed, if we broadened our search. Two websites, Canadian Cancer Trials here at home and ClinicalTrials.gov in the United States, listed ongoing experiments. I expected because the population in the United States was about ten-fold greater than in Canada, our southern neighbor would have a larger selection and be a richer resource.[3] But I didn't know much else: I had no idea how you signed up there, whether Canadians would be welcome, whether it was easy or difficult to get in, or what the costs would be. I was about to embark on an intensive learning program.

Gordon and I decided that I would do most of the trolling for prospects. Once I had identified a possibility, I would turn over the information to Gordon, who would delve into the details. I believed lambro was the best option but was prepared to consider other therapies as well. Lambro was a Merck product, but Bristol-Myers Squibb had an equally promising anti-PD-1 drug in the works, nivolumab. Staying flexible would help us maximize the chance that Gordon would get in somewhere. On ClinicalTrials.gov I found a lambrolizumab study identified as NCT01295827 and open to patients with melanoma. Although this phase I safety trial was in the early stages of testing, registering in it wasn't like jumping off a cliff into the great unknown. Other human beings had gone before and researchers had already published results. The FDA had given it a kind of blessing by announcing it was prepared to fast track acceptance. Joining the study was still gambling, but the prospects of beating melanoma were better with the experimental medicine than with standard drugs. And this trial had a big plus: no control arm. All the subjects received the investigational medicine, albeit according to different schedules and doses.

ClinicalTrials.gov spelled out which patients were eligible for each of the experiments in its database and specified the cities—sometimes as many as a hundred or more—in which they were running. I could also see whether a particular location was "still recruiting"—a key bit of information. In those places, investigators were looking for more people to participate. If a site was described as "active but not recruiting," the study was ongoing but had its full complement of patients. Helpfully, ClinicalTrials.gov provided the postal or zip code of the hospitals or clinics testing a new medicine. Unhelpfully, it omitted the names, addresses, and phone numbers of most of those centers. It usually did not disclose who the chief researchers were either, presumably to reduce the number of calls they received. Nevertheless, I hit upon a stratagem. I probed Google by using the relevant postal codes and the word *melanoma* as a search term. When I did so, Google provided the names of the institutions offering trials I liked. Then I could find their phone numbers. I was in business.

I called Sloan Kettering in New York, Cancer Care Alliance Center in Seattle, Yale University School of Medicine, Providence Portland Medical Center, Pacific Medical Center Research Institute in San Francisco, and The Angeles Clinic in Santa Monica. I soon learned ClinicalTrials.gov was not always accurate. The receptionist at Sloan Kettering told me the lambro trial I wanted, NCT01295827, was closed there, although I could submit Gordon's records to see if anything else appropriate might be available. When I called the clinic in Portland, I heard it had a spot for one person and fifty people on the waiting list for a lambro study. The discovery left me in a state of panic. I felt I was on a sinking ship and the lifeboats were filling rapidly. I e-mailed the patient matching service at Bristol-Myers Squibb in the United States to see if I could turn up something else, and I also rang Merck Canada. Often I wasn't able to reach a live person; I left messages and wondered if I would ever hear back.

I said to Gordon, "It seems so unfair."

He said, "There isn't anyone handing out the fates—anyone who could be fair or unfair." That evening I dissolved:

> *May 23. I lost it. I began crying. I told Gordon how much I loved him, how much love he had poured into the world around him, into orchids and blue poppies, wine-making and photography. I said how much he had supported me in my crazy writing career, how good a father he was. I wept and he hugged me. And then we were sitting on the sofa and I was quieter and Gordon asked me if I would ever feel like playing tennis and I said, "Probably not, but what about badminton?" So after the storm of tears, we played badminton. I lost 11 to 1. We came inside and starting watching a movie, "Shakespeare Wallah" and then halfway through the movie, Gordon began kissing me, and we made love. Afterward, he said, "There's so much emotion washing around." And there is, we ride this great sea of emotion; it's like kayaking over a kelp bed. Sometimes you get stuck, and have to push hard with your paddle, then are released and shoot through a clear bit, and get stuck again, and the whole mass is moving and swaying under your boat.*

May 24. We went for a walk in the Capilano Canyon, a couple of blocks away from our house. On a weekday, the canyon was more or less deserted. We stopped often and kissed under the trees and beside the rushing river.

"I feel normal," I said. "It's kind of weird when you consider what's hanging over us."

"If there is a threat, it makes sense to respond," Gordon said. "But you don't have to respond all the time. You can go for a walk, enjoy yourself, have a good sleep. You don't have to be *on* all the time."

May 28. Dr. Omid Hamid, the director of Melanoma Therapeutics at The Angeles Clinic in Santa Monica, called back, responding to my message. I was stunned to learn he might have an opening for Gordon in the lambro trial that interested us. By now its number—NCT01295827—was imprinted on my brain. I had found only one location for it in Canada—in Quebec—but so far my call was unanswered. If we wanted lambro, the United States seemed the way to go. My fears about overflowing lifeboats receded a bit. Dr. Hamid was a soft-spoken man who carefully explained what was involved in participating. Gordon would have to fax down any reports or letters he had about his case and provide a tissue sample of his original tumor. Then he'd have to come down to Santa Monica for an initial visit, another scan and blood tests. If he met the criteria after all that, he'd be in the trial. "Have Gordon call my assistant, Robert," Dr. Hamid said, "for an appointment, sometime next week." I was elated. *An appointment? Just like that?* I told Gordon about this positive development, but we didn't have much of an opportunity to enjoy it.

May 29. Sharon, my mom's caregiver, phoned to say that my mom "crawled" to the front door to open it when she arrived in the morning. My mom, who was ninety-three, had been living on her own, with some help a couple days a week. When I talked to her, she denied actually crawling, but admitted having trouble walking.

"Did you fall in the night?" I asked.

"I don't remember," she said. "Maybe."

"Should we take you to the emergency room, Mom?"

"No, no. . . . It's not that bad."

Gordon and I were supposed to see Dr. Smiljanic that morning to discuss the options in light of the new PET scan results. I really wanted to be there, and I told my mom that Gordon and I were going to see his oncologist. "We'll come right after," I said, feeling guilty. I didn't know what else to do.

"Sharon is here, don't worry," she assured me.

I'm not worrying, I'm reeling! I thought to myself.

Again, we slipped into our customary seats in the examination room at Lions Gate, and then Dr. Smiljanic apologized for not giving us the report himself. Gordon shrugged. "That's okay," he said. He just wanted to get on with planning. Gordon told Dr. Smiljanic we had been investigating clinical trials. He nodded approvingly: "I've been fighting the BCCA for another course of ipilimumab, but since it didn't work the first time, you might be better off trying something else."

On November 1, 2012, the BC Cancer Agency began funding ipilimumab, but because it was such a new and expensive drug, oncologists had to apply to a committee for authorization. I could imagine that negotiating a second round of the drug might be even more difficult than getting the first. I was glad satisfying the members of that committee was not the only way we could get to one of the newer immunotherapies. I liked having my eggs in more than one basket.

Gordon showed Dr. Smiljanic the sheaf of information we had collected. Our first choice was the lambro study, NCT01295827, but he wasn't as enthusiastic about it as we were. Since it was phase I, less was understood about it. Dr. Smiljanic preferred another option on our list—a nivolumab investigation in Edmonton. This was an open label trial for people who had failed ipilimumab and who would be given either nivolumab or chemotherapy. "Open label" meant that the patients would recognize which medicine they were receiving (chemotherapies and immunotherapies are administered according to different schedules, so once the participants had a timetable, they would know what they were getting). The nivolumab trial was phase III, so further along in the testing than the lambro. For that reason and because the lead investigator was someone Dr. Smiljanic knew and trusted, he was more comfortable going with nivolumab. He said, "I can give you a referral to Dr. Smylie."

The trial had positive aspects, but also a significant downside: "A third of the patients will get chemo," Gordon pointed out.

"That's true," Dr. Smiljanic said. "But there might be a crossover option."

"Crossover?" I asked. "What's that?" The concept was new to me.

Dr. Smiljanic explained that sometimes, if patients were not doing well with the standard therapy, they might be offered the newer drug. This sweetened the bitter pill of randomization—a bit. Drug companies had started to provide crossover because, although the statistical analysis of the results was more complicated, the fact that participants were guaranteed an opportunity to try the new therapy hastened the recruitment of volunteers.[4] Still I could see the solution wasn't perfect. By the time the patients received the investigational medicine, their cancers might have spread and be harder to eradicate. Furthermore, they would be starting the immunotherapy at a disadvantage—weakened by months of disease and the toxic chemotherapy.

"If you are randomized to chemo, do you have stay in the trial?" asked Gordon.

"No, no, of course not," Dr. Smiljanic said. "It's completely voluntary."

"So I could enroll, and then if I got the chemo, drop out?"

Dr. Smiljanic nodded.

"Okay," Gordon said, "I'll try it."

"I'll send a fax to Edmonton. Ideally," Dr. Smiljanic added, "you should be in treatment by the end of June. If we did another scan, I think it would show an increase in the number and size of the tumors."

Dr. Smiljanic's comment just fueled my natural inclination to move rapidly. Clearly, we had to act without delay. Could we swing it?

I left feeling rocky. As Gordon drove over to my mom's, we mulled over the choices again. What was the best way to play our hand? Where did the probability of winning lie? We were gambling—a strange way, I thought, to be choosing medical care.

"If you go with Edmonton, and you end up randomized to chemo, would you drop out?"

"I could, although there would probably be consequences," said Gordon.

"You'd miss out on the crossover option."

"That's right, and it might be harder to get into anything else with Bristol-Myers Squibb."

"And if you went for another trial, you might wind up no better off—in chemo again."

"Well, I could go for a second course of ipi."

"Dr. Smiljanic said he was fighting the BCCA for it. We didn't ask him why he was fighting, but whatever the reason, it's clear we can't count on your receiving it. And I think the numbers are better for the newer immunotherapies like lambro anyway."

"Well then, there's The Angeles Clinic."

"Yeah," I said. We would have to keep both balls in the air—for now, at least until some clarity emerged.

When we got to my mom's, she was obviously in pain. Moving from one position to another was challenging for her. Again, I asked her about going to the hospital, but she shook her head vigorously. She was adamant; she wanted to see her physician, Dr. Julian Ospina at the Pacific Spirit Clinic. So in keeping with her wishes, Gordon, Sharon, and I somehow bundled her into the car and off we went. Dr. Ospina is a charming man who often tells my mother she must have been a beautiful young woman. She blossoms under his compliments. Today, however, he cut the niceties short. Dr. Ospina gave us a requisition for an X-ray. If we could get the imaging done that afternoon, he would probably receive the results the following day. "Will my mom be alright at home?" I asked. "Yes," he said, "if she has twenty-four-hour care." Sharon offered to mobilize her Filipino friends, and I thought we could fill any remaining hours with the help of a care agency I had used before. Somehow we'd manage.

We headed over to the X-ray center. The expedition was trying for my mom, but she didn't complain. Once we arrived, she was whisked into the X-ray room. Being ninety-three has some advantages. As we were waiting, I got a call from Daniel at Cancer Care Alliance in Seattle. I went out into the hall to talk. Fumbling in my purse for a notebook and pen, I realized the only way I could speak on my cell phone and take notes was to sit on the floor. I slid down, leaned my back against the wall, and rested my notebook on my lap. I hoped not too many people would come by. Daniel said that in his center, one lambro trial was closed. But another one was open—for people who had "failed" ipilimumab. I told Daniel that Gordon had received ipi as an adjuvant therapy, but the melanoma had spread anyway. He didn't know whether that would qualify Gordon for this study and asked me to wait a few minutes while he verified. When he got back on the line, he said he was sorry, but the trial was only accepting patients who had taken ipi while they had measurable tumors that grew despite the therapy. I sighed. It seemed crazy to me. Weren't Gordon's six tumors clear evidence of failure? Daniel gave me a phone number of someone else in Seattle who might be able to help, and I thanked him.

We drove my mom home and she collapsed on her sofa, completely worn out. Sharon, who had been on her phone, said she had caregivers lined up for the next couple of days and I thanked my lucky stars for the Filipino village, this deeply connected network of loving and sunny ladies. We would be in sore straits without it. Gordon and I bought a wheelchair and some other supplies that my mom and Sharon needed. Then we drove home and I collapsed on *my* sofa. Later in his diary, Gordon would describe the events as *a hairy week so far.*

The next day I called Dr. Ospina, who told me that my mom had some bad cracks in her pubic bone. She would be fine, however, if someone was with her for at least three weeks. Dr. Ospina promised to visit, and I called my mom's case manager at Pacific Spirit to see what else she might need and what we could rustle up in the way of assistance.

Gordon rang up Dr. Hamid's assistant; he had some questions. Gordon learned that the initial visit would take two days. If he wished, he could have an appointment the following week. The consultation would cost $550, but if he were accepted, the charge would be waived or discounted. Gordon said he would think about it and call back the next day.

Then Gordon phoned Edmonton to see if his referral had arrived. It hadn't. Not yet. Confident that Dr. Smiljanic had faxed off his records, as he had promised, Gordon explained that it must be there. "Could you look around?" he asked. He told the receptionist that this was urgent, that Dr. Smiljanic wanted him to receive treatment by the end of June. She said she would see what she could do. Gordon hung up and said, "I think they consider me a pain-in-the-ass."

"They haven't seen pain-in-the-ass!" I replied, feeling I was the champion in that regard.

May 31. Gordon phoned Robert at The Angeles Clinic again. They talked about details: that Gordon should bring a CD with the last PET scan results and that the BC Cancer Agency should courier off a tissue sample from a recent biopsy. Gordon found out that he had to have an MRI of his brain while he was in The Angeles Clinic, and some blood tests. Robert told him that if he were eligible, he would start treatment a week or two later, and for those visits, a one-night stay would probably be long enough. The therapy would be given every two or three weeks and he might receive it for as long as two years. If he enrolled, he would be flying to California every two or three weeks—not a pleasing prospect, but manageable and certainly better than moving down for the duration. Gordon made an appointment in Santa Monica for noon on Tuesday, June 4.

Then Gordon called Edmonton, and Shelley took his call. She told him that the referral had arrived and that Dr. Smylie would be reviewing it on the morning of June 3. Gordon also asked about crossover and she explained that the trial did provide it. If the results indicated nivolumab was better than the standard therapy, all the patients in the control arm would switch. But, as is so often the case, a snag emerged. The crossover wouldn't happen fast; it could only occur after a significant body of research was amassed. Nevertheless, Gordon chose to postpone his visit to Santa Monica. He wanted to be at home, to get Dr. Smylie's review. The fact that Dr. Smiljanic preferred Edmonton weighed heavily in its favor. And it was in many ways simpler. The flight was shorter—one and a half hours compared to three. It also seemed likely that any expenses associated with being in a trial would be lower in Canada than in the United States. Gordon phoned Robert to tell him what he was doing. Diplomatically, Robert said he understood completely why Gordon might prefer to participate in a Canadian study if possible. And he assured Gordon that a spot would still be available over the next couple of weeks. I was uneasy about giving up what seemed to be our only bird in the hand but, with some reluctance, accepted Gordon's decision.

June 1. I was worrying about my mom. I said to Gordon, "She has suddenly entered into that horrible stage of extreme old age." He wrote in his diary, *Lore is gaunt and frail, forgetful and repetitive.* She'd been a fashion designer, a woman with great verve and style, and I hated to think of her so diminished. But when we visited, I found that her spirits were reviving. She was eating better and so far the household seemed to be functioning smoothly. Progress!

June 2. We needed a break. We drove to Buntzen Lake in Port Moody, about an hour from our house. We started walking in a sun-laden forest thick with moss and proceeded through groves of cedar and Douglas fir trees. We ate our lunch sitting on a small strip of gravelly beach. I remember Gordon looking at the water lapping on the shore. He said,

"Look at the wavelets. They hit the beach and dissipate. But nothing is lost." Believing that he was really talking about himself I said, "You're not a wavelet, Gordon." He said something about me abusing the metaphor—treating it as a relationship of identity when really it was just finding some similarities. I shrugged and smiled. Gordon was being Gordon.

10

IT'S NOT BRAIN SURGERY

June 3. A day of upset and anxiety.

Shelley told Gordon his eligibility for the Edmonton trial was doubtful on one point: no tumors were present when he received the ipi. She was going to check with Bristol-Myers Squibb. *This again*, I thought. It was weird—that a guy who had rampant cancers would be so often tripped up by the lack of them. Shelley promised to call back later in the day or the next with the verdict. As usual, the prospect of negative outcomes loomed large—that Gordon wouldn't be accepted in Edmonton and rejected in Los Angeles too. *Nothing's going to work!* Talia called twice, "Don't panic, mom!" she said. Tom called twice too—once to invite Gordon to lunch.

I kept reading the runes, seeing only mistakes. *Woulda shoulda coulda*. I tormented myself with the idea that Gordon should have had a PET scan as soon as we got the suspicious CT report. Because we went the biopsy route, we didn't get confirmation of the melanoma for another two weeks. We lost an opportunity. And then when we knew about the melanoma, we missed again. If we had stayed home, we probably could have sped up the PET scan. If the BC Cancer Agency was slow to provide, the local private clinic in Burnaby or the Swedish Medical Center in Seattle would have obliged.

About a year before this, we had canceled a trip to Australia. Why didn't we forgo this one? We trusted Dr. Smiljanic when he said "the timing wasn't that critical." Maybe he was right, but I didn't think we'd ever made a mistake by pressing for earlier appointments. As a general rule it made sense. Now the melanoma was streaking ahead again. I berated myself over and over for wasting valuable time, for being complacent, for relying on things to work out, for "living in a fool's paradise." I wrestled with rue and regret, and anticipated the future with apprehension. I felt I was in a place surrounded by black shadows. And, aware that I wasn't the first person to have been there, I began reading "The Inferno":

> Midway in our life's journey I went astray
> from the straight road & woke to find myself
> alone in a dark wood[1]

Gordon took a call from a research coordinator whom I had phoned about a nivolumab study in San Francisco. Based on what Gordon told him, the coordinator thought he would probably qualify. I was puzzled by his assessment. The number of his trial was the same as the one in Edmonton. Why was he more optimistic about Gordon's eligibility than Shelley was? Was he making a mistake? Or was Shelley? No doubt, BMS was exerting control, getting all the clinics to follow the same rules. I didn't think they could have different interpretations. If Gordon was rejected by Edmonton, I thought he would be excluded in San Francisco too. Still we kept the information—in case.

On June 5, I called the National Institutes of Health (NIH) in Bethesda, Maryland, and learned about another kind of treatment called adoptive cell transfer. In one study currently open, T cells were harvested from patients, encouraged to multiply, and then transferred back to combat melanoma. Early research into this technique had shown that if participants were temporarily depleted of their existing immune cells, the transplanted ones were more effective. To prepare subjects for the procedure and reduce the population of native white blood cells, they were given chemotherapy and whole-body radiation. As they were at an extremely high risk of developing infections, they had to stay in hospital for three weeks. When I asked whether the NIH would accept Canadians, I was told that they would, and indeed that travel expenses for both the patient and an accompanying spouse would be paid. It sounded like an eleventh-hour idea to me. I found the fact that the trial was all-expenses-paid disconcerting—a recognition of how unappealing it was. However, I noted the details; I didn't know what we might need.

By the afternoon, we had not heard from Shelley, so Gordon made an appointment at The Angeles Clinic with Dr. Omid Hamid. Gordon wrote an e-mail to Dr. Smiljanic to explain why:

> Dear Sasha,
>
> There have been delays regarding Edmonton. There is still doubt as to whether I qualify for the trial, or am excluded because there was no evidence of disease progression during my course of ipi. As a backup plan, I've booked an appointment with Dr. Omid Hamid in LA next Tuesday (June 11). Dr. Hamid is running a lambrolizumab trial, two arms of which are specific to melanoma.

Gordon requested some reports and Dr. Smiljanic's assessment of his condition. He closed the letter this way: "I hope you appreciate that I need to develop alternatives to Edmonton." At 8:30 that night, Dr. Smiljanic sent an e-mail to his assistants asking them to fax Gordon the documents the next day.

We were on track to get Gordon to the golden-eyed lizard.

The following day, Shelley finally called. The Edmonton study was out.

June 10. Flying to L.A. for my appointment at The Angeles Clinic tomorrow.

Cruising at thirty thousand feet above the west coast of North America, drinking ginger ale, Gordon got out his lined notebook with the black cover. He began to write: I want to get clearer on the psychological reinforcers of self-concern. Why do we think we have a special kind of reason for being concerned about ourselves in the future—a kind that does not apply to anyone else? Gordon was always asking questions that most other people didn't give a second thought. He filled a few pages and then in the late afternoon, the plane touched down in Los Angeles.

Gordon's hotel was just a few blocks away from the clinic so the next morning he walked over. In good spirits, he snapped pictures along the way—of jacarandas, spectacular tropical trees laden with blue blossoms. Later he wrote for his blog, "The clinic was very LA—they share a building with CBS films."[2] After checking in, he was quite taken by how efficiently the U.S. health-care system worked for him. Right away, he was assigned to a "scheduler"—a personage not often encountered in the Canadian system. She arranged a raft of procedures for Gordon to get done in the day and a half that he would be in LA—an MRI, CT, EKG, chest X-ray, blood work, and a biopsy.

But before all the tests, Gordon met Dr. Omid Hamid, who was chief investigator on the trial. He was going to examine Gordon and answer any questions he might have about the study. An ebullient, rather dramatic-looking man with slicked-back hair and a goatee, Dr. Hamid radiated confidence. He told Gordon that the drug he was interested in showed nearly a 50 percent efficacy rate, even in patients who had failed ipilimumab. Subsequently Gordon wrote, "Fifty percent is amazing—like Russian roulette with three chambers loaded. Those are odds I'd jump at."[3] The power of the therapy certainly did seem spectacular, particularly if you compared it to older medicines. The chance they would work was even worse than Russian roulette with five chambers loaded. Dr. Hamid echoed Gordon's enthusiasm for the new treatment. He said, "If I had what you had, I'd break down walls to get this drug." Then he gave Gordon a paper about the results of a recent lambro trial on which he was the lead author. Published on June 2, it was hot off the press. This all sounded very positive, but a hiccup emerged.

After Dr. Hamid examined Gordon, he told him that he would qualify for a lambro trial, Then it turned out that the study Gordon wanted was closed. Another study was open, but unlike the original one, it had a chemo arm, either dacarbazine or P & C (paclitaxel and carboplatin). Gordon had come to LA in the first place because he liked the idea of a no-chemo study, so this news was most unwelcome. But Dr. Hamid told Gordon he had to check something. He left the room, came back in five minutes, and explained that he had alerted the drug company, and they'd kept a slot open for Gordon. So in the end, all was good.[4]

Next Gordon read and signed an eighteen-page consent form. The document noted that when the trial opened, 148 men and women had already been treated with MK-3475 (this was Merck's other, less evocative, name for lambro). The form enumerated four pages of possible outcomes, including death. In lawyer-like fashion, it stated, "The primary purpose of this study is to learn more about anti-cancer agents that may benefit others in the future. There is no promise that the study drug you receive will treat your cancer and that your condition will get better. It might stay the same or it may get worse. The drug you receive may even be harmful." (Of course, death is rather harmful!) It also pointed out, "You may leave the study at any time without penalty." Gordon's participation was voluntary all along the way—just as we had assumed.

Unconcerned by the caveats, Gordon signed the papers without hesitation and went on to have some blood tests. That evening, he phoned me to say it had been touch and go, but he was in. He got the last slot. "Dr. Hamid thinks you're a great advocate for me. He said I should buy you a diamond ring." I laughed. "I don't need that! If you get better, that's ample reward."

At 2:00 a.m. the next day, I woke bug-eyed with fear. I was afraid that something nasty would scotch Gordon's participation. What if he had a brain tumor? It was an exclusion criterion, a reason for disqualifying Gordon on this trial and on many others.[5] Mind you, I had no reason to suspect a brain tumor. Gordon had no neurological symptoms—no headaches, no tremors, no numbness, no tingling, no difficulty moving. But I ruminated anyway.

That morning, while I was eating breakfast, trying to dispel my night terrors over coffee and toast, Gordon walked past the jacaranda trees to a scanning facility. He reported for an MRI and then strolled back to The Angeles Clinic to have his remaining tests. A technician took some blood samples while preparing Gordon for another scan, a CT, and told Gordon he was going to see what other blood work needed to be done that day, so that he could draw all the tubes from the same IV. "I was impressed by his proactive efficiency," Gordon wrote. When the technician returned, he said that someone would be coming to speak to him. This was the first hint of a fly in the ointment. Shortly, Dr. Hamid appeared, removed the IV, and led Gordon to another room where a group of people were reviewing his scan.

"That's your brain." Dr. Hamid said simply. Someone had drawn a green box around a small area on the side of Gordon's right cerebral cortex. The box was annotated with the measurement, 1.7 cm. "Unfortunately the MRI found a tumor in the brain." Dr. Hamid said, "You need to fly home, have that surgically removed, and get some radiation. Then come back here and we'll get you into another trial. The operation looks straightforward because the tumor is on the surface. It isn't brain surgery," Dr. Hamid said. Then he paused a moment and remarked, "Well, actually it is." Gordon laughed, appreciating the gallows humor.

But as Gordon prepared to leave the building, he was rattled. The investigative whirlwind had spun to a halt. He no longer knew what was expected of him. Awkwardly, he asked Dr. Hamid, "Is that it? Do you need me for anything else?" Dr. Hamid shook his head. The clinic, which could schedule a variety of complex procedures in the minimum amount of time, had no protocol for this. Melanoma had reared its ugly head. The black tumor was back, scattering Gordon's hopes and anticipations in its wake, and trampling his plans underfoot. Everything had changed. A green box encircled a black spot and that was it. Gordon went across the street to a Mexican restaurant for lunch and called me from there. "Are you sitting down?" he asked. When I heard the question, I caught my breath. I grabbed a stool. "Yes, I am now. What happened?"

"The MRI I had this morning found a brain tumor."

"Oh no!"

"That disqualifies me for the trial. Dr. Hamid said I have to go home, have the tumor taken out and then have radiation. After that, I can come back down to LA and get into another trial."

"It's such rotten luck."

"There were some more tests I was supposed to have tomorrow morning. But now they're canceled. So I'll try and get an earlier flight."

"That would be good."

"I'll let you know how I do."

"I love you."

"I love you too."

I hung up. Devastated, I thought back to my blue moment at 2:00 a.m. How did I know? Sitting on our old kitchen stool, elbows on the counter, head in my hands, I brooded about the effort we had expended over the last three weeks. All for nothing. All those phone calls—for nothing. Dr. Hamid had said Gordon could get into another study, but I wasn't reassured. So many things could go wrong. By the time Gordon had the surgery and radiation, Dr. Hamid's trials might be full. Besides, the brain operation didn't do anything about Gordon's other six tumors. Untreated, they would probably grow; they might multiply, move into vital organs. Dr. Smiljanic had said Gordon should be having a systemic treatment by the end of June. Now we had no chance of reaching that target. I remembered that when Gordon got a second lump on his arm I thought, *Game over*. Our current situation was even more so, if that was possible. We had come so close and now were staring at the brink. I wondered how much of the summer we would be able to enjoy.

A couple hours later, Gordon phoned. "I got the flight changed. I'll be in Vancouver around ten tonight."

"I'll meet you at the airport."

"You don't have to do that."

"I'll be there. I want to be there."

I phoned the kids and we arranged to meet for dinner at a small Japanese restaurant near Tom's place. Once there, I told the waitress I couldn't make a choice. I was under too much stress. "Would you please pick for me," I said.

Gordon e-mailed Dr. Smiljanic from LA to give him the news. And then he caught the Vancouver-bound plane. His familiar black notebook was with him as usual:

> *June 12. Dr. Hamid recommends surgery, followed by radiation. After that—and a four week wait period, he could perhaps offer me another anti-PD-1 drug trial. That one, of course, might have a chemo arm. Or there could be another brain tumor by that time. It may be that the odds have got too long, making further resistance futile. Surgery has a cost, which I don't know. RT [radiation therapy] of the brain would have a cost too, which I also don't know yet. These things remain to be assessed.*
>
> *I don't know where to concentrate my efforts. If I can't cure this brain melanoma, I can't finish the book—there's a good year or more of work left. I can write posts. I could make some videos. Or I could just spend time with the people who love me. The last thing I want to do is neglect them. Those are the deepest connections.*
>
> *All the important things that would go in my book are in my blog, although not said well enough for many people to understand. We humans need to learn how to spread our concern more widely. When we learn that, not only will we be happier, we'll be incomparably more effective.*

When I got to the arrivals area, the overhead screens told me that Gordon had already landed. I didn't have to wait long before I saw him striding through the door to the lounge. We hugged and I kissed him, under his Indiana Jones hat. He smiled and we walked out, hand in hand. The situation wasn't good, but at least we were together.

I I

THE FIRST HILL

I don't remember when we had The Conversation—probably in the morning over breakfast. Maybe along with grapefruit, coffee made from freshly ground beans, eggs, toast, my home-made jam. I don't know who started it, but I do recall that I was deeply influenced by a story of Atul Gawande's that I had read a few years before in the *New Yorker*. Called "Letting Go," it described some of the "heroic measures" that doctors take to prolong lives—doomed remedies that can make patients' last days utterly wretched. I was haunted by Gawande's account of Sara Monopoli, a young woman diagnosed with lung cancer in June 2007.

After she had four rounds of chemotherapy, each one more experimental than the last and each equally ineffective, the cancer kept progressing. She developed a malignancy in her thyroid and then brain metastases. A week of radiation left her completely fatigued. She lost weight, coughed up blood, experienced nausea and dry heaves. One morning in February 2008, when she was struggling desperately for breath, her husband took her to the emergency room. The doctors diagnosed pneumonia and prescribed antibiotics. They wanted to put her on a catheter and talked about using a ventilator to keep her breathing. Finally, her mother put an end to it. She thought her daughter had suffered enough. "*No*," she said, "You aren't going to do anything to her."[1] Sara died shortly afterward. As Gawande writes:

> This is a modern tragedy, replayed millions of times over. When there is no way of knowing exactly how long our skeins will run—and

when we imagine ourselves to have much more time that we do—
our every impulse is to fight, to die with chemo in our veins or a tube
in our throats or fresh sutures in our flesh. The fact that we may be
shortening or worsening the time we have left hardly seems to register. We imagine that we can wait until the doctors tell us that there is
nothing more they can do. But rarely is there *nothing* more that
doctors can do. They can give toxic drugs of unknown efficacy, operate to try to remove part of the tumor, put in a feeding tube if a
person can't eat: there's always something. We don't want anyone—
certainly not bureaucrats or the marketplace—to limit them. But
that doesn't mean we are eager to make the choices ourselves. Instead, most often, we make no choice at all. We fall back on the
default, and the default is: Do Something. Is there any way out of
this?[2]

Neither Gordon nor I wanted his life to end in such a miserable fashion.
You shouldn't make difficult decisions when you're at the end of your
rope. The time to think about end-of-life scenarios is while you're still
feeling good, in command of your faculties. Writing in his journal, Gordon had already considered the possibility that his chance of surviving
was remote: *It may be that the odds have got too long, making further
resistance futile.* Had we reached that point? I didn't want Gordon to
fight on, just for me, to suffer on my account. Would it be better if he
concentrated on living the next few months—as fully as possible?

  According to Gawande, some seriously ill patients who chose hospice care lived longer than those who elected to continue with treatments. He wrote: "Curiously, hospice care seemed to extend survival
for some patients: those with pancreatic cancer gained an average of
three weeks, those with lung cancer gained six weeks, and those with
congestive heart failure gained three months. The lesson seems almost
Zen; you live longer only when you stop trying to live longer."[3] I certainly did not want to shorten Gordon's life in a vain effort to find a
cure. Maybe the brain metastasis was It—the signal to let go. On the
other hand, maybe it wasn't. Did it make sense, as Dr. Hamid advised,
to seek further therapy? As we pondered these difficult questions, we
concluded that we needed more information. On the morning of June
13, Gordon sent Dr. Smiljanic an e-mail:

Dear Sasha,

On reflection, I'm wondering whether the course of action Dr. Hamid recommended, outlined in my e-mail to you yesterday, is the best one. Obviously, this brain metastasis is a serious development. The surgery sounds feasible. The post-surgical radiation could be done too, but I wonder about side-effects and what it would buy me. What are the chances of being able to pull off the scenario Dr. Hamid recommends: surgery on the tumor, RT, then a wait period, then another MRI to qualify me for another anti-PD-1 drug trial? Is whole-brain RT effective against local recurrence—i.e., another brain metastasis? I guess all that would take longer than 2 months. What are the chances of the tumor load in the rest of my body reaching a point that the odds of a good response to the immuno-therapy becomes vanishingly small?

My goal is to use the time remaining to me well. I don't want to waste it pursuing heroic interventions that face impossible odds.

I'll try to make an appointment to see you soon.

All the best,

Gordon

Meanwhile I e-mailed Kathy Barnard a message along the same lines as Gordon's: "No one has told Gordon how long he has to live, but, of course, I have seen the stats. I am wondering whether it is better to think about how to spend the remaining months in the best way possible, or whether it is realistic to continue pursuing treatment. Any ideas you have would be welcome, of course."

Kathy invited me to call, which I did. A few years ago, she said, a brain metastasis *was* the end of the road, but no longer. Treatments were better and people were living longer. She recommended we look into Gamma Knife surgery. It wasn't available in Vancouver but was offered in Winnipeg at the Health Science Centre there. When I searched for it on Google, I learned that Gamma Knife surgery was a minimally invasive procedure used by neurosurgeons to treat benign and malignant tumors. A website about the service in Winnipeg stated: "The Gamma Knife delivers a single high dose of ionizing radiation emanating from 201 cobalt-60 sources. The highly focused beams of gamma rays are guided with surgical precision, without a scalpel and without the usual risks of open neurosurgery."[4] Individually, Gamma Knife rays emitted minimal radiation and caused little collateral damage as they traveled to the cancer. Tissue was destroyed only where they all converged, at the tumor site. Apparently, most patients returned home the day of the surgery and resumed full activities within one or two days As usual, after my conversation with Kathy, a sense of possibility energized me and I phoned Winnipeg to see whether Gordon would be a candidate for radiosurgery. The possibility looked fairly likely, but we would have to send over his records to get a definitive answer. The next day we heard from Dr. Smiljanic:

> Hi Gordon,
>
> I am very sorry to hear about the brain metastasis. I personally have had two patients with MM and brain mets go into a long term remission with surgery, RT, and then Ipi. In your case it would be a pd-1 drug. I would strongly encourage you to move forward as Dr. Hamid suggests. Nothing worsens the quality of life more than rapidly progressive cancer, especially in the brain.
>
> We will meet soon to discuss.
> Sasha

We weighed the pros and cons of surgery. If Gordon did nothing, his condition would deteriorate; if he had the brain metastasis removed, he might improve significantly. The excision required a hospital stay and would cause some discomfort. But afterward, Gordon could try an anti-PD-1 drug. Although these medications didn't help everyone, by all reports they carried a low risk of debilitating side effects. With Dr. Smiljanic's and Kathy's encouragement, we resolved to go on. We were convinced we shouldn't give up just yet, and that another surgery (Gordon's sixth!) was worthwhile.

But first we had to deal with an immediate problem—the tumor was flexing its muscles, making its presence felt. When Dr. Hamid had shown Gordon the MRI of his brain, he had pointed to a small black spot. This was the cancer. Around it was a cloudy white area that took up about a quarter of the right hemisphere. Dr. Hamid explained this was where the tumor was exerting pressure on the brain. Although Gordon had experienced nothing unusual while he was in Santa Monica, at home his head began to throb and the fingers of his left hand ached—an effect of that pressure. He managed to get an appointment with Dr. Smiljanic—for the following week on Monday. To alleviate the pain he was experiencing, Gordon went to the outpatient clinic at Lions Gate Hospital. A resident prescribed dexamethasone, a corticosteroid, to reduce the inflammation. She correctly predicted that the drug would act quickly and Gordon would feel better soon.

The long-term picture was still unclear. But Gordon was taking that in his stride. As he wrote:

> *Sunday, June 16. We've been talking about the odds of my dying sometime soon, perhaps within the year, perhaps before next summer. My attitude towards myself is different from my attitude towards Claudia. I said to her, "I don't feel as though I would be cheated of the rest of my life." I can easily imagine feeling that way, though. A few years ago, I think I would have felt that way. That's self-concern. In the same vein, I can imagine starting to eat a bowl of raspberries, like the one I had this morning—so delicious—and feeling cheated if I thought it would be my last bowl of raspberries. As if that would somehow diminish the deliciousness of this bowl. I can imagine a patina of regret and sadness, suffusing my experience, and robbing it of its savour. But I don't feel that way. I wholeheartedly enjoyed my raspberries, I enjoyed going shopping, I'm enjoying writing this. Most things I do, feel like putting out seeds, like our old maple does every fall. A few, precious few, fall on fertile soil and sprout. Most of them die in the spring, because I mow them down or weed them out. One or two may get away, maybe, and start a new maple tree! I think my seeds' chances are better than that.*

Gordon seemed more concerned about me than himself, figuring that I might have the harder row to hoe:

> *I love Claudia and she loves me. She is afraid of being lonely. Of course, she will not be alone, but she will not have me to hold her and kiss her neck and make love to her, and to have the long conversations we have. I'm sympathetic, the more so when I think of how I would feel if I were to lose her. Death is a loss. She said that if I don't feel cheated of the rest of my life, she shouldn't feel cheated of it either. That's true, I think, but the cases lack symmetry. To be the survivor is to have a bigger problem. Right now I have a problem too, but I know how to face it—pursue my doctors assiduously, be realistic about the chances of various interventions working, consider the intervention/non-intervention trade-offs. To face the problem of adjusting to life without the loved partner—that is a much more difficult prospect, fraught with uncertainty. I think it's a path one can only approach by setting out and finding one's way. It cannot be pre-*

planned very well. I would like to spare her the grief and the loneli-
ness and, especially, despair. I know she'll be surrounded by love—
immersed in love (which is the way I feel all the time these days)
supported by the kids, who are so warm-hearted, and by many other
friends, and by people she hasn't met yet. Claudia, you know I'm
with you for every step.

The following morning, we were both sitting at Lions Gate Hospital in
an examination room, in our usual positions. Gordon asked whether
radiosurgery was a good idea, but Dr. Smiljanic explained that in a case
like his, "regular" surgery had better outcomes. Apparently, if the brain
metastasis was easily accessible, as Gordon's was, and if a patient had
only one or two tumors, the current protocol favored the physical knife.
The Gamma Knife was reserved for cancers deep in the brain that a
neurosurgeon would have difficulty reaching. Dr. Smiljanic said he
wanted to arrange the surgery as soon as possible. He was going to
phone Dr. Ramesh Sahjpaul, a neurosurgeon in North Vancouver, right
away. Then he would book a consultation with Dr. Kim-Sing to discuss
the postoperation radiation.

"Why don't you go for coffee?" suggested Dr. Smiljanic. "Come back
in half an hour or so and see what I've been able to do." He was
accelerating the process. I liked that! We didn't go for coffee; we went
for a walk around the hospital. The sun was shining, the sky was blue,
and the June flowers were bursting forth in the residential neighborhood. We drank in the warmth and pleasure of the day. When we got
back, we learned that Dr. Smiljanic had wrought a wonder. "You have
an appointment tomorrow morning at nine," he said.

The next day, we were in Dr. Sahjpaul's office. We were first in line,
and we realized he had squeezed us in ahead of what was probably
already a packed schedule. A tall, handsome man, he was also kind, and
explained everything he was going to do in detail. He had an air of quiet
competence that I found reassuring. He told us that Gordon's operation
was called a "craniotomy" because he would remove a piece of the skull
to get at the tumor (and put it back of course). Then he took out a sheet
of paper and drew a picture of Gordon's brain. The cancer was on the
right side, in a part of the brain called the parietal lobe. It abutted a
sulcus—one of the brain's grooves, or furrows. Dr. Sahjpaul said he had
one concern—the malignancy was also close to some blood vessels. He
hoped to be able to peel them back and preserve them before extract-

ing it. The procedure would take about two hours and carried a slight risk of seizure, but in general it looked straightforward. Gordon would spend two to four days in the hospital to recuperate.

"When can you do it?" Gordon asked.

"Probably later this week on Friday, in the afternoon. We'll confirm that. "

"Here at Lions Gate?"

Dr. Sahjpaul nodded. I was delighted with our progress and felt Gordon was well looked after.

"I liked him," I said, as we walked down the hallway.

"I did too." Gordon smiled.

On Thursday, Surgery Eve, we went on a romantic date—dinner at Blue-Eyed Mary's, a restaurant in West Vancouver. We pledged not to talk about metastatic *anything*. We sat across from each other at a small table. I looked at Gordon's dark blue eyes, warm and friendly. He told me he was happy and that he felt bathed in love. Actually, he told me this quite often.

But that night, I didn't sleep well. Neither did Gordon. I kept contemplating the impending operation. What if it caused a bleed? What if Dr. Sahjpaul couldn't get the melanoma out because of its proximity to blood vessels? What if another brain metastasis cropped up before Gordon got the radiation that was supposed to "sterilize" the brain? What about the possibility of cognitive impairment from either the cancer or the treatment? What if no trials would accept Gordon? What if there was no immunotherapy for him? What if Gordon died? We'd already had a conversation about this and I remembered our voices:

"We all die," Gordon says.

"Later is better than sooner," I say.

On Friday morning, I drove Gordon over to the hospital and then came home where I met the kids. They were going to keep me company so I wouldn't go stir crazy. We had lunch, walked in the nearby canyon, played cards, and then returned to the hospital. The procedure was over sooner than I expected—a good sign probably. When we got to the neurology ward, we found Gordon was awake. His head was wrapped in gauze and he looked like a wounded soldier, but he felt not bad. He had been reading. He told us that Dr. Sahjpaul was pleased with the operation. Everything went well. We played cards for a while and then left him to his hospital dinner. It wasn't much postop, but we promised to bring something better the next day. On Saturday, I was giving a writing workshop, so the kids took over; they visited, entertained Gordon, and ensured he had a good dinner.

On Sunday morning, I arrived at the hospital with our waffle-maker, batter, yogurt, maple syrup, local strawberries, and a big thermos of coffee. After Gordon showed me an outdoor patio where we could sit, I found a plug, set everything up, and we had breakfast, overlooking North Vancouver and the sea beyond. We could see the freighters in Burrard Inlet looking like a child's toys in a bathtub. Gordon was eager to come home. "A hospital," he declared, "is no place for rest and recuperation." He hadn't been able to get much sleep the previous night. The lady in the bed next to him had been trying to escape. She'd wait until the nurses were occupied with another patient, grab a wheelchair, and using it as a walker, head for the door. This would trigger an alarm the nurses had set up; they would catch her and bring her back to bed, where she would wait intently to make another run for it.

A physio, who dropped by to take Gordon for a walk up and down a couple flights of stairs, took in our domestic arrangements, smiled, and said, "You probably don't need me." "I've already tried the stairs," Gordon told her. When a nurse came in to take Gordon's vital signs, he asked when he would be discharged. "I'll get Dr. Sahjpaul to call you," she assured Gordon. Meanwhile, she gave me instructions about how to change the dressing. Earlier Gordon had written about looking like Frankenstein's monster when he had a few staples in his arm. Now with the staples in his head, the resemblance was even more striking.

All in all, I was surprised by how well Gordon was doing. Soon Dr. Sahjpaul was on the line; he talked for a few minutes and determined he had no reason to keep Gordon in hospital any longer. After discussing medication, he mentioned a follow-up appointment in a couple of weeks. I was amazed brain surgery could go so smoothly.

Gordon saw his recovery as hiking over a series of hills without any maps. The terrain was challenging; still he was committed. Turning back was not an option but whether he would reach the final destination was also in doubt. The first hill was the surgical removal of the tumor. That had been handled—quite expeditiously. He got over the hump in less time than he expected he would need. The second was the radiation therapy to avert another melanoma in the brain. At this point, the second hill was shrouded in mist. Finding the right path was going to be hard. The trails crossed and criss-crossed, petered out, or ended in a briar patch. Gordon needed to remain mindful that he could easily get lost. The third hill was getting into a clinical trial for an anti-PD-1 immunotherapy drug. This goal was way off in the distance—blue and shimmering. Gordon had no idea how he would get to the top. He could only hope that once he got nearer, the way might seem obvious.

12

BECAUSE I AM AN OPTIMIST

Gordon, his head still swathed in a gauze turban, was lying in a hammock we have strung up between two walls in our living room, next to the front windows. I was sitting on the sofa and a stack of papers lay on the coffee table between Gordon and me. Highlighters in hand, we were deep into radiation studies, marking important passages and trying to assess which route was best. We were planning the second ascent. We didn't have much time. On July 8, Gordon had an appointment with Dr. Kim-Sing; he wanted to be prepared—to understand what the alternatives were.

In the first half of the twentieth century, physicians could do nothing for patients with brain metastases. By the early 1950s, however, they were starting to treat the entire brain with radiation to relieve pain and extend life—a little. Prakash Chinnaiyan relates that two decades later, this was the standard therapy for cerebral metastases.[1] And then in a 1990 landmark study of patients with only one tumor, Roy Patchell showed that if surgery was performed before whole brain radiation therapy (WBRT), results improved significantly.[2] In Patchell's trial, the median length of survival for participants who had surgery and radiation was twice as long as for those who had radiation alone. This sounded like an encouraging advance, until I realized that the median length of survival for that first group of patients was a mere forty weeks—not even a whole year. When I thought about that, I got depressed. I decided the only way to stay sane was to try to find the best program we could, and not think too much about the amount of time it was buying us. I knew that researchers had been plugging away to make progress. More than twenty years had elapsed since Patchell wrote his paper, and I expected survival had inched up since then.

Actually, it turned out that better life expectancies were creating a new problem. Whole brain radiation seemed to be associated with long-term cognitive deficits of various kinds, including memory loss. When patients were living for only a few months after treatment, you didn't have to consider what might emerge down the road. But now with improved prognoses, possible future developments mattered. One confounding factor was that the research into the effects of whole brain radiation was not as clear cut as you might wish. As Gordon writes, "These studies fail to distinguish deterioration due to WBRT, from deterioration due to other causes. Other causes include the brain cancer itself (a problem shared by everyone who gets WBRT), cancer in other parts of the body, chemotherapy and other medications, other radiotherapy, and prior neurological disease (strokes and such). So, we know that brain deterioration follows WBRT, but we do not know how much of it is *caused* by WBRT."[3] The picture was murky, in other words, but we knew enough to be wary.

By the mid-1990s, physicians developed the ability to hone in on brain tumors with radiation and obliterate them, leaving the surrounding healthy tissue more or less unscathed.[4] This was called stereotactic radiation surgery (SRS), even though no incisions or cuts were made. More recently, oncologists offered targeted radiation as an adjuvant treatment when cerebral metastases had already been excised surgically—to reduce the risk of further metastases. Using a Gamma Knife or similar technology, they aimed only at the area from which a tumor was removed—the part of the brain where recurrence was most likely. They were hoping that stereotactic radiation therapy (SRT) would preserve brain function while prolonging life. How well did this work? The approach didn't seem to be associated with memory loss. Intriguingly, a 2009 study of forty-three patients showed that those individuals who received local radiation after surgery lived longer than those who had whole brain radiation.[5] Obviously, larger clinical trials were needed to confirm the finding.

Some doctors continued to use whole brain radiation but experimented with ways of mitigating its possible negative effects. One idea was to make adjustments to spare the hippocampus—an important region for the laying down of memories. Another was to give patients a drug called memantine, which alleviates some of the symptoms of Alzheimer's.[6] Researchers were looking at radiosensitizers, medicines that increase the vulnerability of tumor cells to radiation therapy. Investigators were also experimenting with hyperbaric oxygen therapy (HBOT) to improve the cognitive function of patients receiving whole brain radiation. During HBOT, patients breathe pure oxygen in a pressurized room or chamber. A well-established therapy for decompression sickness, a hazard of scuba diving, it is approved in Canada and the United States to treat wounds that won't heal as a result of diabetes or radiation injury. But the studies into using the technique to ameliorate whole brain therapy, though positive, were hardly definitive.

I was out of my depth. We could search the Internet for additional articles and studies, but would that help? I felt dazed by all the information we had so far unearthed. How could we find our way? Then I had an idea. "Why don't we go down to Seattle with a list of questions?" I asked Gordon. "We can get a second opinion—pay to talk to an oncologist. It will be a crash course in Radiation 101." The chief advantage of going to the States was being able to speak to a physician for an hour or so—much more time than we'd ever get up here. Gordon liked the proposal, began searching for an expert, and hit upon Dr. Vivek Mehta, the director at the Center for Advanced Targeted Radiotherapies in the Swedish Cancer Center and a leading light on radiation in the Seattle area. I phoned the center and asked if Gordon could have an appointment with Dr. Mehta. "Is July 1 okay?" the receptionist asked. "Yes," I said, surprised that I was able to get a booking so readily. I remembered that we had gone to Seattle a year ago, almost to the day. An anniversary of sorts, then. When I asked about the price, I was pleasantly surprised again. $135 US. *Not too bad,* I thought, *for an hour with a consultant.*

Gordon wrote to Dr. Smiljanic to tell him of his plans. He was in agreement: "A second opinion is never harmful; as well, it is likely good timing to see the Seattle doctor first." Our trip to the States would not delay or obstruct anything that might happen at home.

June 25. Last night I felt overwhelmed by the forces arrayed against us. Gordon said, "What forces? It's only the melanoma." Yeah, right, I thought.

A few days before, I had e-mailed Kathy Barnard asking whether she knew anyone who had personal experience with whole brain radiation. She provided a number for Shannon Gaudette, who lived in the Fraser Valley. Gordon called right away, but it took a few days for him to connect because Shannon was out of town. When they did finally speak, Gordon met an astonishing woman. Shannon's battle with melanoma was old, stretching back eight years to 2005 when she had a small mole on her right arm removed. It was positive for the skin cancer. Five years later, she developed a lump under her arm and her lymph nodes were taken out. In May 2011, when Gaudette, thirty-nine, was pregnant, her dreams of starting a family were seriously imperiled. She started having difficulty walking and then her husband, Brad, found her collapsed in the shower. He took her to a local hospital, where an emergency MRI revealed that the melanoma had metastasized again—this time to Shannon's brain. Two large tumors—one the size of a lemon and the other the size of an orange—were the cause of her problems. A doctor told Brad he might be able to keep Shannon alive long enough to deliver her baby. But Shannon was only twenty-four weeks along in her pregnancy. At this age, the baby might survive but it was chancy. The situation for Shannon was dicey too. Then an obstetrician came up with another idea—send Shannon to Royal Columbian in New Westminster, the oldest hospital in British Columbia, famed for its trauma care and neurosurgery. It could handle a brain operation and a high-risk neonatal delivery at the same time, if that was necessary. In an ambulance, with lights and sirens blazing, Shannon was whisked off to Royal Columbian. By then, she was completely incapacitated, drifting in and out of consciousness. Dr. Richard Chan, a neurosurgeon, told Brad that the cancers had to be taken out right away, but he could not guarantee that Shannon would be able to walk or talk afterward. As Brad watched her being wheeled away to the operating room, he had no assurance he would see her alive again—or that their baby would be born safely. Dr. Chan removed the tumors in a six-hour, high-risk operation, and the baby stayed safely in the womb. When Shannon came to, she had some difficulty using her legs and arms, but she could talk. Soon she began to walk normally again and, remarkably, gave birth to a healthy girl, Madeline, in August. Not long after, under Dr. Kim-Sing's supervision, Shannon had two weeks of whole brain radiation at the BC Cancer Agency— to prevent a relapse. She reported no recurrence of the cancers and did not notice any long-term negative effects from the radiation. When Gordon said he would be seeing Dr. Kim-Sing to discuss radiation, Shannon told him, "I think Dr. Kim-Sing is brilliant. I would trust her with my life. When you see her, tell her I say 'Hi.'" Gordon said, "Of course."

I was inspired by Shannon—by her determination to do whatever was necessary to be a mom to her little girl. Her courage helped me face what lay ahead. Maybe terrible forces weren't arrayed against us after all. Perhaps Gordon was right about that. I was also impressed with how Shannon's medical team pulled her through what seemed to be a calamitous situation. I felt that Gordon and I might be lucky too. I was still fretful, but I had hope.

We drove south on a hot sunny day. I was glad Gordon was no longer wearing the bandage on his head. I thought it might have caused the border officials to look at us askance. Gordon still had the metal staples embedded in his skull though, and it seemed a fortunate coincidence that they were on the right side. The guard wouldn't see them, unless, for some reason, we had to step outside the vehicle. That horror-movie-look might have aroused suspicions also. We crossed the line without incident.

At the Swedish Medical Center, we found ourselves in the same airy, light-filled lobby where we had waited for Gordon to have his PET scan the previous year. I opened my diary: *Usual somatic symptoms, heart racing, stomach tension. Deep breath, that helps.*

Dr. Mehta ushered us in to a small windowless conference room. We shook hands and sat down. I glanced at Gordon, who looked unruffled, even though we were on the cusp of a momentous decision. A great deal was at stake. Slipping into a student role, I looked at Dr. Mehta expectantly. First, he gave us some background. He said that years ago, it was rare to see just one brain metastasis, but now because of better CT and MRIs (and more frequent use of them) finding solitary lesions was not uncommon. These single cancers were more likely in melanoma patients than in other cancer patients. He told us that an idea once quite prevalent, that melanoma was radiation-resistant, was a myth. Melanomas have a range of responses to radiation; some are very resistant, others not at all. The myth grew out of older studies that included biased data.[7] But he also mentioned that radiotherapy seemed to work better with melanomas if delivered in fractions of 5 Gray or higher[8] (since 1975, a Gray, a measurement unit named after British physicist Louis Gray, has been used to quantify the radiation a patient receives). I wondered if the oncologists who noticed "radiation resistance" had been unknowingly underdosing their patients.

Gordon had a sheet of questions, to which he now turned. He began by asking, "Do you think that I should skip the radiation and just move on to an anti-PD-1 trial? That would get me to a systemic treatment faster." Both Gordon and I were cognizant of Dr. Smiljanic's recommendation to start the drug treatment by the end of June. We were now past his deadline and we had no clue how much danger Gordon was courting as a result.

Dr. Mehta shook his head. "Observation alone is not a good option. Forty-five percent of patients who don't have follow-up radiation after surgery, relapse at about a year."[9]

We could scratch that choice off our lists.

"How good is stereotactic radiation at preventing recurrence?" was Gordon's next question.

"Unfortunately the data on cavity radiation is not the best," said Dr. Mehta. "A recent study showed its benefits, but the patients may have been cherry-picked to confirm the researchers' biases. However, there is one clear advantage to it. It takes less time to complete treatment— just one to three sessions—compared to whole brain radiation."

"How good is whole brain radiation?" Gordon wanted to know.

"It's important to realize that while the risk of recurrence is reduced, it doesn't drop to zero. Afterward, there still is a possibility of developing additional brain metastases."

"And how solid is the evidence on cognitive decline?"

Here Dr. Mehta concurred with what Gordon had been able to discover. "The data for cognitive decline following whole brain radiation is weak because controlled studies have not been done to sort out how much cognitive decline is due to radiation, and how much is due to cancer, chemo, or preexisting conditions."

"We read," Gordon said, "several suggestions about preserving intellectual capacity following whole brain radiation. I was wondering what you thought about these ideas. For instance, I saw that some researchers have proposed making adjustments to avoid the hippocampus."

"That sounds like a good idea, but I don't know much about it."

"What about memantine? It's a drug used in the treatment of Alzheimer's," Gordon said.

Dr. Mehta nodded. "We haven't used it here, so I can't really comment on that."

"And then we saw something about radiosensitizers—to make the tumors more susceptible to radiation."

Dr. Mehta smiled. "Radiosensitizers? They've been talked about for decades at oncology conferences, but nothing much has come of them."

"Okay," said Gordon. "What about hyperbaric oxygen treatment (HBOT)?"

Dr. Mehta wasn't encouraging on that score either. He told us that tumors were more resistant to radiation in a low-oxygen environment. So increasing the oxygen levels in the blood should theoretically make it easier for radiation to successfully eliminate the cancers. He was, however, skeptical about the ability of HBOT to increase blood oxygenation.

As I saw it, some things were now clearer. The strategies we had been seeing about mitigating the effects of whole brain radiation were unsuccessful, experimental, or unavailable in any practical sense. If we opted for whole brain, we wouldn't find much in the way of amelioration. Our choice was between stereotactic and whole brain (unvarnished). It still wasn't certain to me which was best.

"Dr. Mehta," I asked. "What would you do if you were in Gordon's shoes?"

"Whole brain," was his answer, followed by a thoughtful pause as he looked Gordon over. "But in your case, the argument for stereotactic becomes more compelling."

"Why is that?"

"Because I'm an optimist and would like to believe that the MRI showing just one tumor was correct." I recognized his way of thinking—the assume-the-contract-can-be-made approach. If the best scenario was correct, there was no need to risk the possible damage of whole brain radiation. But it was high-stakes poker. If we were right, we'd win big, and if we were wrong, we'd lose big.

Dr. Mehta told Gordon that if he were interested in having SRT at his center, he should talk to Dr. Chris Loiselle, the best person to explain the specifics. Then Dr. Mehta left us with one last thought. "If you do have SRT here, it would be preceded by a high-resolution, thin-slice 1-mm MRI. This would give comfort if it turned up nothing new. If it did turn up something, you would be treated with radio surgery at the same time as you had the SRT." The original MRI in Santa Monica was not nearly as finely grained—5 mm, the standard slice. The Seattle scan would be able to pick up smaller lesions—though not any microscopic ones.

We shook hands, thanked Dr. Mehta, and promised to think about what he had said.

July 2. Still in info-gathering mode. I don't feel too bad. Neither does Gordon.

Gordon wrote Dr. Smiljanic a long e-mail summarizing all he had learned from the conversation. He concluded by writing: "I tend to lean toward the SRT option, as I really don't like the idea of causing cognitive damage. (I'm writing a book.) However, I recognize that the worst damage is likely to be caused by additional brain mets should they occur. Can you offer any guidance? I will contact Dr. Hamid to get his take on it, particularly with respect to the consequences should I start another anti-PD-1 trial and then discover another brain metastasis."

"Hi Gordon," Sasha wrote back. "Your final point is exactly the one I would focus on . . . the implication of further brain mets on your ability to carry on with the PD-1 trial. Other than that, I will have to let the radiation oncologists duke things out."

Gordon wrote to Dr. Hamid the same day as well, asking for his opinion.

"I would go with SRS here," Dr. Hamid wrote back, "as it saves you the risk of long-term morbidity. Also the fact that the lesion was so big and there were no others makes me think that this is a solitary lesion without other smaller ones below the limit of detection lurking. Get your SRS and then we can speak in regard to open options."

This had started out as a fifty/fifty proposition. But now stereotactic seemed to be gaining favor among the doctors we were consulting. When, following Dr. Mehta's suggestion, Gordon spoke to Dr. Loiselle at the Swedish Medical Center, he said that if he were in Gordon's situation, he would choose stereotactic for himself. The deciding factor for him? Less damage to the brain.

I myself was still leaning toward whole brain. Though stereotactic was better at "local" control, whole brain was more likely to keep "distant" metastases in check. When I told our son, Tom, what I was thinking, he said, "Mom, you probably have enough information to regret whichever decision you make."

"You know me too well!"

On July 8, we were once again at the BC Cancer Agency, our final fact-finding mission with Dr. Kim-Sing. She arrived with a resident, introduced us, and then said to Gordon, "You look very well, for someone who just had brain surgery."

He flashed a wide grin.

She reminded Gordon that the situation was grave. "If we do nothing, the likelihood of recurrence is about 80–90 percent." She was putting the odds of failure even higher than Dr. Mehta had, but we were already convinced that observation-only was not a viable approach, so the grimmer statistics didn't change anything. "Whole brain radiation will bring the risk down to 30 percent," Dr. Kim-Sing explained. "The plan would be for 30 Gray in ten fractions—half from the right side of the brain, half from the left."

"How does that dose compare with the radiation I had under my arm?" Gordon asked.

"At that time, you received 48 Gray over twenty fractions."

"When could you start?"

"Today. We could start now." I understood that Gordon could walk out, go down the hall, climb on a radiation bed, and begin. He would go home with an irradiated brain. I trembled slightly. It was a little like being in *One Flew Over the Cuckoo's Nest*. I know it wasn't the same, but there were unnerving analogies.

Gordon still had some issues he wanted to settle. He told Dr. Kim-Sing about the studies we had been reading and about our trip to Seattle. He posed the same questions he had asked Dr. Mehta, about strategies to protect the brain from radiation. Dr. Kim-Sing was not any more positive than Dr. Mehta was. She told us that the BC Cancer Agency was proposing a small study to look at the effect of shielding the hippocampus during radiation but there were no results yet, and Dr. Kim-Sing wasn't recommending the practice. As for drugs to preserve or protect brain function? They weren't approved either, and she wouldn't be considering them. She explained that although the agency did stereotactic surgery to remove tumors, it did not provide any stereotactic adjuvant therapy. So standard whole brain radiation was the only option on offer.

"Is there any good reason I might not know about why I shouldn't have stereotactic?" Gordon asked.

"If you go to Seattle," Dr. Kim-Sing pointed out, "you will have to pay for it. Can you afford that?"

"It's pricey, but manageable, about $22,000."

"Well," she said, "if you can swing it, maybe that's best for you. Later if you need whole brain therapy, you can always come back."

As we got up to go, I remembered Gordon's promise to Shannon. As we walked out the door, I said, "We told Shannon Gaudette we would be seeing you, and she said to say, 'Hi.' She's quite amazing, isn't she?"

"She's just great!" Dr. Kim-Sing beamed. "She's my favorite."

Dr. Kim-Sing's "blessing" had tipped the balance. Gordon was inclined toward stereotactic anyway, and now I felt reasonably comfortable with the choice too. As soon as we got home from the BC Cancer Agency, Gordon phoned Seattle. "I'd like to make an appointment." We gathered up various scans and reports for the doctors he would see and made preparations to be out of town for a couple of days.

The die was cast.

On the morning of July 10, Gordon had his thin-slice MRI at the Swedish Medical Radiosurgery Center. Afterward, we spent a couple hours walking around Seattle. I took photographs of weather-beaten houses, old roses in tangled weedy gardens spilling over fences. The neighborhood had an amiable, worn seediness about it. We came across a Vietnamese restaurant, Ba Bar, and wandered in for lunch. The food was fresh-tasting and zesty. But once the main course was over, I (uncharacteristically) didn't want any dessert. I was on edge, anxious to get back for Gordon's appointment with the radio surgeon. We were supposed to get the results of the MRI and discuss the procedure that would take place the next day.

I was apprehensive because, as I reminded Gordon, "Lately, all the scans and tests have been worse than expected."

"But a couple of lumps you fretted over in 2012 turned out to be harmless seromas."

"I think I'm developing a phobia anyway."

Thanks to my anxiety, we got to our 1:30 appointment well ahead of time. We were waiting to be called in, when Tom phoned and asked me how I was. I said, "Scared shitless, but otherwise okay." And then I laughed. "What else is new?" Tom asked. He laughed too.

Trying to derive strength from their sangfroid, again I recalled the airmen who were fighting in the Battle of Britain, facing horrendous casualty rates. How did they manage when what lay ahead was so grim? The pilots didn't fall to pieces, they got in their planes, got airborne, and returned or didn't. Maybe the secret was to dial back your imagination—stop scaring yourself with mental pictures of your future self. But that was hard for me. My mind's eye was particularly active when it came to those visions of me and my loved ones. It was both a gift and a curse.

Gordon's appointment began with a nurse, who briefed him thoroughly. She took pains to describe in detail how his head would be immobilized during the upcoming procedure. Gordon wrote, "I would have a metal frame screwed into four points of my skull. The pain would be managed by local injections of lidocaine; but the lidocaine itself would sting at first. I'd be given dexamethasone against inflammation, and Ativan to keep me calm. After the frame was attached, I'd have a quick CT scan." The purpose of the scan was to locate the target area of the brain in relation to the frame. Once its coordinates were established, they could be used to direct the gamma rays toward the target. The frame helped to orient the knife and also kept Gordon's head rigid, ensuring that the target didn't move. "This precise spatial registration would allow the Gamma Knife to work with sub-millimeter accuracy," Gordon explained, "zapping only the thin margin of the surgical cavity and nothing beyond. The whole procedure would last about four hours. I could listen to music if I wanted. I would probably go to sleep."[10]

By now we knew the drill when it came to results. Only physicians give you results, technicians and nurses never do. Nevertheless, Gordon could not help himself from asking the nurse who was explaining all this to him, "Did the MRI show any surprises?" In a departure from routine, she shook her head and said, "From what I overheard of the doctors' discussion, I don't think so." The tension drained out of my body, ebbed away.

Next up was the radio surgeon, Dr. Sandra Vermeulen, who was directing the therapy. A blonde woman with a friendly smile, she was an accomplished researcher as well as a clinician. Her website listed multiple research papers on a variety of topics. She had experience with different radiosurgical techniques and several types of tumors. First she said, "The MRI showed no new hot spots." Naturally, I was greatly relieved to hear this. Dr. Mehta's optimism was justified! Getting confirmation of a solitary tumor was one piece of evidence that we had come to the right decision. Then Dr. Vermeulen gave us another. For melanoma, she noted, a cure was more likely with a higher dose of radiation. Since stereotactic could be delivered in bigger fractions than whole brain radiation, it seemed to her the better choice.

"You can have a look at the MRI yourself," Dr. Vermeulen offered. "I'll put the disc into my computer." As we leaned forward to see more clearly, she pointed at the area that needed to be treated and commented, "Your surgeon did a good job." I peered intently at the black and white image, but I couldn't see why she said that. In truth, I didn't know how a good job would look different from one that was mediocre. But, of course, I was gratified that she admired Dr. Sahjpaul's handiwork, bearing out my trust in him. Dr. Vermeulen went on to compare the new MRI with the one Gordon had at The Angeles Clinic. Off and on, we had been concerned about a mass it had revealed in his right parotid gland. This is a salivary gland—one of two located in front of each ear. In the scheme of things, it was not a big priority, just one of several tumors! But Dr. Vermeulen informed us that in the new MRI, the lump was the same size as it had been previously. "It's probably not melanoma," she concluded. "If it were, it would have grown." More relief.

And then she pulled up the results of Gordon's PET scan from May; we were getting a pretty extensive tour. "You have six tumors," Dr. Vermeulen said. The PET scan showed what was going on below the neck, and Dr. Kim-Sing had already told us about this. Nothing new there. But what Dr. Vermeulen said next did surprise me. "The tumor in your buttock is quite aggressive, but those in your pectoral muscle and on your chest wall are less so." I knew that PET scans detected metabolic hot spots. I hadn't grasped that they revealed a range of suspicious activity. Radiologists obtain SUVs (an acronym for "standard uptake values"—not a type of car) for different regions in the body.

They are a measure of the amount of radioactive sugar that tissues absorb. Because malignant tumors grow quickly and need more energy than normal tissues, they will have a higher SUV. Any number over 2.5 indicates a cancer is likely; the higher the number the more probable a malignancy is. The tumor in Gordon's buttock had an SUV of 14 and indeed the PET scan reported it had grown .4 cm since measured in a CT scan five weeks before. But the melanomas on Gordon's chest wall and in his pectoral muscles were pegged with SUVs of 2.6 and 3— rather indolent tumors. Dr. Vermeulen cheered me up considerably. She made me feel that the melanoma was not the implacable enemy I had imagined. All of the lumps were clones of the same mutated cell and I did not expect them to behave differently. Learning that they did was like suddenly realizing that not all of an invading army's divisions were equally bellicose. To someone who has had no experience of metastatic melanoma, this might seem like cold comfort indeed. Gordon still had six cancers in his torso—six tumors that had not been treated and might spawn others. But I was grateful for what I saw as positive indicators. Hope does not require a large foothold to gain purchase.

Gordon told Dr. Vermeulen that after the Gamma Knife procedure, he was going to look for a systemic immunotherapy. She nodded approvingly and said that if it did not shrink all of the remaining tumors, he could have more stereotactic radiation to mop up the residue. Not with the Gamma Knife though—with a CyberKnife. She explained why by giving us a mini-lecture on the difference between the two complementary technologies.

By now we understood that to keep the Gamma Knife on target, Gordon's head had to be kept rigid. But if you had cancers in your torso, the Gamma Knife would not work. Patients need to breathe and you can't keep them perfectly still. The CyberKnife is able to cope with this challenging environment, however, by continually taking images of the patient's body and adjusting to small changes in position. If necessary, tiny gold pellets, markers called fiducials, are placed at strategic locations to help guide the CyberKnife. The Swedish Medical Center had a CyberKnife, but Dr. Vermeulen assured us that there were a few in Canada too. "You could probably have the radiation done at home." I liked her can-do attitude—her view that Gordon had problems, but not overwhelming ones. Even if immunotherapy was not entirely successful, we could take steps to respond to the situation. During her three-quarters of an hour with us, Dr. Vermeulen answered all our questions, including the critical one: "How many of these do you do?" "About two a day," she said, and promised various follow-ups as part of the deal. We felt our money was well spent.

After nearly two hours of talking about scans, tumors, and radiation, we needed a walk. We drove to Discovery Park, at the northwest edge of Seattle—five hundred acres of parkland, home to many birds and marine mammals. As he got out of the car, Gordon spotted a swing on a long rope. He hopped on, and for several minutes whooshed through the warm dappled afternoon light. We approached a cliff overlooking Shilshole Bay and Gordon took some pictures of the ocean. Then we had dinner at Toulouse Petit, a New Orleans–style restaurant. Gordon wrote, "It was like a date night."

Unexpectedly, it was a good day. I felt confident we had done the right thing. I had no regrets.

Gordon and I were staying at a hostel-type hotel attached to the Swedish Medical Center. It wasn't fancy, but it was convenient, so it only took about five minutes to walk to the radiation clinic. Gordon and I reported at 6:30 a.m., as requested, and then I went back to our room, where I was going to read until I heard that Gordon was being discharged.

Downstairs, Gordon was given a local anaesthetic and a sedative. As advertised, the frame (sometimes called a halo) was attached to Gordon's skull with pins, two on his forehead and two at the back of his head. The pins were shaped like nails with a screw thread on their heads. As the pins were screwed into the frame, Gordon could feel them turning and digging into his skull. This hurt, Gordon wrote, "but not for long. Then it felt like a hat—a metal hat that was way too tight. Touching the frame produced the odd sensation that it was part of my body, as though I'd grown antlers or an exoskeleton. If anything touched the frame, the noise sounded very loud." After Gordon had the CT scan to guide the gamma rays to the radiation target, a helmet with hundreds of holes in it was placed over the frame. These holes provided additional focus for the gamma rays. The helmet locked onto a couch, which then slid toward the Gamma Knife where the treatment actually took place. When it was done, the team offered to take a picture of

Gordon. He agreed and posted the result on his blog. In it you can see
the silver metal pins denting Gordon's forehead and a silver metal bar
obscuring his mouth. He labeled the shot "Me trying to smile with a
metal frame screwed into my skull."[11]

I got a call around 10:30 and returned downstairs to meet Gordon.
He was instructed not to drive (one of the reasons I had come along)
and was given a report on the operation and a disk with the MRI. "The
MRI came to a whopping 43 GB,"[12] Gordon wrote. (This was the equivalent of the data in about 14,000 books.) I drove home to Canada.
Later, in the evening, Gordon insisted that he was well enough to at-
tend a committee meeting of his photo club. The members were planning a major competition, which they would host next year. I drove
Gordon to West Vancouver and he happily participated in the discussions while I went for an evening walk along the sea. I was thinking
about next steps. The way ahead was clearly challenging. Later Gordon
would describe it this way:

> The second hill wasn't as arduous as I expected, and I still feel rea-
> sonably fresh. Surveying the third, I don't have a clear sense of dis-
> tance; and there are clouds around the peaks. Nor do I know the
> depth of the valley separating the ridge I'm on from the next upward
> slope. When making plans for my future self, I like to think of him in
> the third person. It makes more than a grammatical difference; it
> helps me maintain an even-handed attitude (commonly called *per-
> spective*). I think about *him*, a guy a lot like me—quite likeable
> (although sometimes maddeningly thick), someone who can be
> trusted to look out for the people I love, a guy whose politics I
> approve of—whose days may turn out much better or worse depend-
> ing on what decisions I make now. Indeed, his life may depend on
> my decisions, so I take them seriously. I feel affection towards him,
> and want things to go as well for him as possible. As for Claudia, and
> for my children and other people I know.
>
> So I peer across the valley, trying to plan his route. The bits of
> slope I can make out look steep. There is too much cloud. I don't feel
> confident he'll make it to the top—find a trial he qualifies for. I must
> assume he can climb the mountain. I know it has at least two peaks.
> If he is eligible for a clinical trial, it is likely to have more than one
> arm. Patients in one of those arms will get old-style chemotherapy.
> That peak is exposed, bleak and dangerous. The other peak holds
> more promise—a mountain hut, with a stove and firewood and

canned goods, where he could take shelter and recover strength—
that is, anti-PD-1 immunotherapy. It's obvious which peak he should
aim for; but I can't tell him which direction to go. And of course,
even if he makes his way to the right peak and finds the hut, he can't
stay there forever. The territory that lies beyond remains unknown: a
50 percent chance of a gentle descent into a friendly valley, and a 50
percent chance of barren terrain and ever-worsening conditions.
How to advise him? I will try to find out more. He will have to pick
out much of the path as he goes along. The trail is poorly marked. I
wish him well. [13]

I would have liked to spend a day taking it easy, but I felt I didn't have
that luxury. Tomorrow was July 12, almost two weeks past Dr. Smiljanic's "deadline." I had to be swift. I planned to get up early and get on
the phone.

13

WE HAVE TWO SLOTS LEFT

Staring at my computer screen at 8:30 in the morning on the day after we returned from Seattle, I took stock. During the past few weeks, while we were thinking about radiation, I had already made some calls about immunotherapy trials. I had learned that sites in Encinitas and Fresno and at the University of California Los Angeles had nothing for Gordon. But Dr. Hamid had welcomed Gordon to contact his clinic again. I also knew that the Beverly Hills Cancer Center had a lambro trial for which Gordon might qualify and that the nivolumab study we had considered earlier was still open in the Melanoma Center at the University of California San Francisco. These last two trials, however, had chemo arms—which was not optimal. Could we find an immunotherapy trial without a chemo arm? Were there any spots left in the lambro trial Gordon had tried to access earlier?

So far, my method of searching for clinical studies had been laborious. Once Gordon and I identified a promising trial, I would use Google to find the name and phone number of a sponsoring clinic. I'd call. Try to connect with the appropriate person. If not available, leave a message. Then I might or might not hear back. All in an effort to learn whether, in fact, the site was accepting new patients. *There had to be a better way*, I thought. I was aware that obtaining a space in a trial we liked was going to be difficult. The slot that had slipped through our fingers in Santa Monica was the last one Dr. Hamid had available; spots elsewhere would be scarce as well. If we were going to uncover that needle in the haystack, I needed to be more efficient.

It struck me that Merck must have a list of the lambro sites that were still open. Confident that someone in the company would be able to give me that information, I phoned the head office in Kenilworth, New Jersey. (The street address was 2000 Galloping Hill Rd., yet another kind of hill to populate our metaphorical landscape. We had the first, the second, the third, and now the galloping.) I was directed to a woman at the National Service Center, which matches patients and trials. She surprised me by saying that while she could give me the names of clinics running lambro experiments, she couldn't say which ones were taking on new participants. (I couldn't tell whether she didn't know or for some reason wasn't allowed to reveal those facts.) She also said that even though she could provide the names of people I should contact and their direct lines, she wasn't able to mention more than three at once.

"Okay," I said. "I'll take what you can give me." Accepting her offer would save me a little time. "What states do you want?" she asked. I paused a moment before replying. I already had phone numbers for clinics in California and had called several of them. Another state would give me information I didn't already have. Texas had MD Anderson, so I said, "Texas," and then I remembered the Mayo Clinic in Rochester— also famous—so I said, "Minnesota." I got names of people to contact regarding trials at the Mayo Clinic, at MD Anderson in Houston, and the START (South Texas Accelerated Research Therapeutics) clinic in San Antonio—a city I associated with the legendary Battle of the Alamo but not advanced medical research.

While I was learning about these prospects, Gordon sent Dr. Hamid an e-mail. He told him that the radiation went well and that a fine-grained MRI showed no evidence of cancer. "I think your recommendation of SRS was a good call!" he added, and asked, "Can you offer me an anti-PD-1 trial?"

Then working from the list I got from Merck, I left a message for Dr. Wen-Jen Hwu at MD Anderson. I contacted the Mayo Clinic where a receptionist took down details about Gordon. After assigning him an identification number, she said she would look over a list of trials in progress at her clinic and call back within five days to let us know what she had found. Finally, I called START. I called it last because I had never heard of it and because San Antonio was the site farthest from Vancouver; getting there involved a two-leg journey lasting about six hours. I spoke to Isabel Jimenez, the patient referral coordinator, and told her about Gordon—that he had melanoma and was looking for an immunotherapy trial. "Do you have a study that's still recruiting?" I asked.

"Yes," she said, "we have one for MK-3475."

"Is it NCT01295827?" I asked.

"I'm not sure," she said.

"Is it the trial with several arms? A, B, C, D, . . . and so on?"

"Yes, that's right. We have two slots left in arm B."

Two slots left! We have to get cracking. I gave Isabel a brief history of Gordon's situation and she said he sounded like a fit. "Can I fax you Gordon's medical records?"

"That would be a good idea. Guillermo Espino, the study coordinator, will look at them and determine whether your husband is eligible."

"How long will it take?"

"A few days, you will hear back at the beginning of next week."

I hung up. Gordon, who was also in the office at his computer, looked at me expectantly.

"I can't believe it, Gordon. I think we might have it—in San Antonio, of all places!"

"Are you *sure*?"

"Well, the coordinator didn't seem to be familiar with the Clinical-Trials.gov number, but her study sounds the same as the one we were seeking. It has several arms; I believe it's the trial you tried for in LA."

"There's no chemo arm?"

"I don't think so."

"But there is a problem—only two spaces left." I glanced at my watch. It was 10:30. "We better get your records faxed off."

Working quickly, we assembled the scan reports, blood tests, doctors' letters, notes on Gordon's previous immunotherapy infusions. We put together a package that was fifty pages long; it grew fatter each time we sent it. At 11:20, I fed the sheets through our aged fax machine, one by one. The device balked and jammed if I tried any kind of mass transmission. The paper rattled through at our end and I hoped it was ratcheting through at the San Antonio end as well, over twenty-two hundred miles away.

We were keeping several irons in the fire. On July 15, Gordon followed up on his e-mail to Dr. Hamid by leaving him a phone message.

The oncologist running the nivolumab trial in San Francisco called and encouraged Gordon to apply. He told Gordon he would need to come to San Francisco for an initial consultation and that he should bring a tumor tissue sample with him as well as a disk with a recent MRI of his brain. He also explained that at his center most costs would be covered by Bristol-Myers Squibb, the trial sponsor. Gordon made a tentative appointment to visit on August 8.

The next day, Gordon left another message with Dr. Hamid. In addition, he spoke to Robert at the Beverly Hills Cancer Center to keep that possibility simmering by letting him know the results of his most recent MRI. In the afternoon, Gordon spoke to the START clinic about the financial arrangements, which were not as advantageous as in San Francisco or at The Angeles Clinic. Merck would pay for the drug, but we would be responsible for scans, blood tests, and the consultations with the doctor. Perhaps, I thought, this was why START still had two slots in its trial; the expense was a barrier that reduced demand. Like the other clinics, START also expected us to cover the travel, although it did have an agreement with a local hotel to give its patients a favorable rate. A welcome break, the discount didn't offset the fact that the airfare to San Antonio was higher than to the other clinics we had been considering. The cost of Gordon's participation in a clinical trial was not our biggest concern, but I didn't want us to pay more than we needed to either. I wondered whether the Medical Services Plan of BC, our government health care, would help us out, since Gordon had run out of treatment options here. I made a mental note to investigate. Then just before dinner, we heard back from Dr. Hamid, who apologized for not phoning earlier—he had been out of town. He confirmed that the trial Gordon had been contemplating in June was now unavailable. He had another lambro study though. This one had three parts: two lambro arms in which the drug was given at two-week and three-week intervals, and one chemo arm.[1] Chemo patients would cross over to lambro if their cancer progressed—was 25 percent worse—after twelve weeks.

"But chemo doesn't work," Gordon said, remembering the dismal statistics on death rates of melanoma patients treated with chemo.

"I have a patient who's doing really well on it," said Dr. Hamid.

One patient, Gordon reflected.

"I'll think it over," Gordon told him.

The following day, Gordon wrote to Dr. Hamid and asked him to send a consent form for the trial they had discussed—lambro versus chemo with a crossover option. He hoped to finalize things with START but was reluctant to burn any bridges.

On July 18, Isabel verified that the START trial was the much-desired NCT01295827 six-part lambro trial. There was, indeed, no chemo arm. The study offered two possibilities—treatment with the investigational drug every two weeks or every three weeks. This was just what we hoping to hear, but then Isabel gave us an alarming revelation. She said Merck had stipulated that all participants should be in treatment by August 9; after that date, it was closing the trial. This posed some serious scheduling difficulties. According to protocol, Gordon couldn't receive any drugs until he had gone through a four-week "washout" following his radiation on July 11. The first day he could have an infusion was August 8, a Thursday. Isabel told us that that unfortunately, START only did infusions on Mondays. The first Monday after August 8 was August 12—four days past Merck's deadline.

Somatic symptoms up the wazoo. Stomach knotted. Heart pounding.

Later in the day, I felt a little better. Gordon talked to Guillermo, who said, "No show-stoppers, so far." He was going to check with Merck about the deadline and said we should hear something the following week.

Gordon wrote,

> *July 20. I definitely feel the buttock lesion again. It is . . . what? Discouraging? No, I'm not discouraged. Sobering? Yes, but that doesn't quite do it justice. It makes me very aware of being in a race against time. What's most uncomfortable is not having much more influence over what will happen. The cards will fall as they may.*
>
> *Went swimming at Whytecliff—always therapeutic! Swimming in the ocean is one of the great pleasures of summer—then climbing on a rock and warming in the sun. A primeval pleasure that takes you right into the present moment. We came home and had steelhead on the BBQ with fresh dill, boiled potatoes with butter, and fresh raspberries from our own canes.*

In a week, we had made progress, but it wasn't solid. If Gordon had another brain tumor, all the trials were off—San Antonio, Santa Monica, and San Francisco. I was already thinking about a plan B. I found a group at Stanford directing a trial of ipilimumab plus radiation for people with brain metastases. I decided to inquire about it—a reconnoitering mission.

> *July 23. Heard from Guillermo this morning—Merck agrees to start the infusion on August 12. Now all I need to do is arrange an MRI to show my brain is clear of new mets!*

At 10:00 that morning Gordon wrote to Dr. Smiljanic: "I am provisionally accepted into a lambrolizumab at START in San Antonio, TX: Aug 5 consultation, first infusion August 12. START asked me to get an MRI done here before I go down. Can you arrange this?" That afternoon, Dr. Smiljanic responded, "Will do."

The weather was stunning. A Pacific high had descended on the coast. The skies were a deep aqua and the sea beckoned. We decided to slip in a week-long family vacation on Bowen Island, only a twenty-minute ferry ride away from our home. Because it was close, Gordon could pop back to the mainland for his MRI, and Tom's wife, Leanna, who was teaching at Simon Fraser University, would be able to make her classes. We were looking forward to getting away from the city when a hurdle developed. On Thursday, the 25th, the day before we were to leave, we still had not heard from Lions Gate Hospital about the MRI. Gordon phoned the imaging department and learned that it had not received Dr. Smiljanic's requisition. Without that, nothing would happen. Gordon then called Laura Wilson. Her official title was Symptom Management Nurse, but her actual role went beyond that. She was a person we had come to treasure for her ability to stir a sluggish bureaucracy into action. Laura said she would probe the matter and then called back to let us know the order had just been sent out. She also reported that urgent cases were waiting a month for MRIs and nonurgent ones, up to two years. She suggested Gordon give the department a day to see if it could fit him in.

When I heard this, I said, "They'll never be able to squeeze you in, if urgent cases have to wait a month. We better go to the private MRI clinic." I had already made inquiries and knew that North Shore Imaging had availability on July 29 and 30. But of course, we still needed a requisition. For some reason that I didn't understand, the MRI department at Lions Gate would not fax its order over to North Shore Imaging. If we wanted an order to go there, it had to originate from Dr. Smiljanic. Since he was in his office that day rather than in the hospital, I suggested to Gordon, "Let's go over, walk the contract."

I was referring to an idea we had first encountered when Gordon was working for a small high-tech start-up company. After several anxious dry months with no orders, the salesman finally closed a major deal with a U.S. customer. Various people had to sign the contract, and to conclude this final step, the salesman flew to Chicago. He said he was going to "walk the contract," take it personally from department to department, to get all the needed signatures. He accomplished in a couple of days what easily might have taken two weeks without his solicitous attention. I always thought the story contained a valuable life lesson, although I never had occasion to use it before.

Gordon liked my proposal, so we went to Dr. Smiljanic's office. When Gordon explained to one of the two receptionists what we wanted, she said we should go back to the hospital for the form. Then Gordon pointed out that he couldn't wait until next week, when Dr. Smiljanic would be back in the hospital. He was trying to get into a clinical trial in the United States and needed an appointment for a scan by Monday or Tuesday, so he could take the report with him to Texas. I added that we already had a requisition, we just needed a copy of it for the private MRI clinic. At that point, the second receptionist offered to help. "I can get that," she said. She found a form, rubber stamped it and told us she would fax it over to North Shore Imaging.

"No, no," Gordon remonstrated. "*We'll* take it to North Shore Imaging."

"You want to do that?" the receptionist asked.

"Oh yes," Gordon said. "It's only a couple of blocks away." We ambled over, stood in line, and got an appointment for Monday 11 a.m.

Bowen. We were staying a place called Ocean Light, overlooking the Salish Sea. Gordon wrote, *It is well named, for it has many windows and is filled with the light of the sky.* We were there to swim, walk, cook, eat, and play games.

July 29. 9:44 a.m. On Bowen Island ferry to Horseshoe Bay.

The morning was glorious and despite having to leave our retreat for a few hours to have his MRI, Gordon was in high spirits:

> *Flags snapping.*
> *Hair flying.*
> *Sun-gleam from the white-painted railing.*
> *A jocund morning!*
> *On the Queen of Capilano.*
> *Now approaching the dock.*

The next day, back on Bowen, Gordon and Leanna hiked up Mt. Gardener—a long trek, seventeen kilometers, with an elevation gain of about seven hundred meters. As they ascended through meadows and forests, they talked about many things—Leanna's work on economic and evolutionary biology, the benefits of meditation, and the relative merits of meditation versus Phantom Self–thinking for mental health and adaptive function. They talked about Tom and about love. At the end, they were rewarded with spectacular views of Howe Sound and the Sunshine Coast.

While Gordon and Leanna were rambling companionably, I was brooding: *The fax with Gordon's results will be at home when we arrive. NS Imaging wouldn't email it to us. It is not how it does things. I dread going home. I will let Gordon read the fax and tell me what it says. My knees will be weak. My heart will pound, my stomach will flutter—as they do just now thinking about it.*

Three days later back in North Vancouver, contrary to my expectation, we found no fax, just a recording from San Antonio requesting results of the MRI. Gordon left a message with North Shore Imaging, asking what had happened, then decided to drive over to the clinic and pick up the report. I was getting more and more nervous, beset by the full suite of somatic symptoms, when I noticed a letter from the MRI folks in our mailbox. I hailed Gordon as he was starting the car, and when he came back into the house, handed him the envelope. I could not bear to look at it myself. We sat down on the sofa, my head buried in Gordon's chest, a coping strategy I used to get through the scary bits in movies. As Gordon read aloud, I was on the verge of panic. I feared a repeat of what had happened in Santa Monica—Gordon being accepted into a trial and then rejected at the last minute due to another brain metastasis. I could hardly comprehend what I heard, but I grasped the upshot: all okay. Gordon faxed the report to San Antonio. I sighed with relief.

August 4, a Sunday, Gordon's day of departure, was not an auspicious day to be traveling. The U.S. Department of State had announced that twenty-five embassies throughout the Middle East, North Africa, and Southeast Asia would be closed due to the threat of a terrorist attack. We thought the airport would be a zoo but tranquility reigned. Perhaps some people had canceled their travel plans. In any case, Gordon whisked through security. While waiting for take-off, he wrote some notes about George Price, a population geneticist whom he had discovered in Oren Harman's book *The Price of Altruism: George Price and the Search for the Origins of Kindness*. Price wanted to understand how altruism could have evolved, a question that also intrigued Gordon.

Meanwhile, at home with my diary, I wrote:

> *Tom says that unless he leads an absolutely quiet life, very low activity, he gets symptoms—fatigue and headaches. I'm going to work on his "case" next week. He says, "There are so few options." It breaks my heart to hear this!*
>
> *Sometimes I wonder if we're crazy chasing all over the continent. Is there hope? I guess we must think there is, or we wouldn't do it. But is it sane to think this? Our wonderful weather is back, but I feel flat.*

> *August 5. My mom and I keep having these weird conversations.*
> *Mom: Gordon has these little . . . little . . . little . . .*
> *Me: (in an exasperated and loud voice) TUMORS!*
> *Mom: What will happen if he does nothing?*
> *Me: Gordon will DIE (also loud and exasperated). I feel my mom keeps making me repeat and repeat these unpleasant facts. It feels like she is tormenting me but I know that's not it. It's more that she needs (likes) to have information repeated and repeated. She said she was sorry for repeating these questions. She caught my distress.*

I tried to remind myself that my mom was ninety-three years old and her mind was not what it once was. But she was still engaged. She cared for us and even though she struggled, she wanted to understand what was happening. I resolved to be more patient but I was aware that my anxiety was an impediment.

In San Antonio, the day was hot, reaching a high of 104° F; the breeze ruffling the leaves in the mesquites and stirring up dust in the scrubby grass brought little respite. Gordon's hotel, in the Medical Center district, was just about half a mile from the START clinic, so he decided to walk. He chose a path that followed the shortest possible route between the small patches of shade along the way. The clinic was in a modern, four-story beige building; its waiting room was spacious and comfortable and the staff, welcoming. Gordon was assigned a scheduler who would make sure he had tests and scans on the appropriate dates. Then he met the director of clinical research at START, Dr. Tony Tolcher, who would be his physician throughout the trial, if he were to be accepted.

A genial man, Dr. Tolcher turned out to be a transplanted Canadian who had grown up in West Vancouver. He went to medical school at the University of British Columbia but moved to San Antonio in 1998 to take a position at the Cancer Therapy Research Center. Later when I spoke to him on the phone, he explained why he left. "For a young person who is ambitious, Canada has a lot of limitations. I just didn't see my career developing as I thought it should if I stayed." He also told me that he had wanted to be a doctor since he was four years old. At first, he thought about being a GP because being a generalist appealed to him. But his plans changed when he was thirteen and his father was diagnosed with lung cancer. He said, "I went into medical oncology because of my father—no doubt about that. I had some unfinished business with this disease, you might say."

Dr. Tolcher has made it his personal mission to get the latest cancer therapies to people who need them. He is impatient with unnecessary "process" that gets in the way. "I always like to tell the story," Dr. Tolcher said, "that in 1998 when I went to work at the Cancer Therapy Research Center, there was one president and two vice presidents. When I left in 2007, there was one president, one executive president, and thirteen vice presidents. They built this enormous administrative structure. It was robbing the institution of much needed resources because each vice president comes with a salary of $200,000. They were essentially falling deeper and deeper into debt." Dismayed by the top-heavy organization that didn't improve the lives of patients, Dr. Tolcher founded START with three other physicians. He wanted to be part of something that was nimble and much more responsive to people's needs. Dr. Tolcher said that because many institutions have complicated procedures that need to be completed before clinical trials can get up and running, "in the U.S. only 5 percent of all patients go on clinical studies." Dr. Tolcher wanted to change how things were done—"to disrupt the standard operating of business."

When Gordon arrived at START, lambro was beginning to develop a name for itself as a "miracle" cure. It made a big splash at the annual June meeting of the American Society of Clinical Oncologists (ASCO), where the *ASCO Post* reported on its "durable" and "significant" antitumor activity.[2] *Nature* followed with a piece called "Immunity Let Loose."[3] The *New Scientist* published an article titled "Skin cancer 'cured' by waking up T-cells,"[4] and its story described tumors completely disappearing. The popular media also paid attention: *USA Today* titled its story "New drugs brighten outlook for melanoma"[5] and told readers that drugs like lambro "can keep cancer at bay a long time." Dr. Tolcher took pains to point out to Gordon that although the medicine had potential, only about a third of his patients would respond. He said, "One of the things you learn very early in life is that you don't overpromise to anybody." Of course, he wanted to help each one of his patients, but he couldn't, at least not with current therapies. Unfortunately, he did not have a reliable way of predicting who would benefit. All he (and the patients) could do was watch for the scans and see what they revealed. In the afternoon, Gordon was going to have a baseline CT. If he was admitted into the study, a second scan at twelve weeks would show whether he was heading toward success or failure.

Another uncertainty revolved around how long Gordon would be in the trial. When he asked what would happen if his tumors disappeared, Dr. Tolcher said, "We just keep going until you can no longer tolerate the drug." Gordon later wrote:

> That is something that happens, sooner or later, to those who are helped by MK-3475. They develop symptoms of "wasting"—fatigue accompanied by weight loss. This is presumed to be an auto-immune response caused by the over-active T-cells. There is no more cancer to attack, so they start in on healthy tissue. When the "wasting" starts, patients are taken off MK-3475 and given steroids to calm the immune system. This reverses the "wasting" process. So far, clinical experience suggests that patients keep their gains against cancer. Every so often, when you're part of a clinical trial (especially if it's

Phase 1), you're reminded that it is, after all, a medical experiment. As long as patients can tolerate the drug, doctors continue administering it because they don't know when it's safe to stop. Better a treatable episode of "wasting" than a recurrence of cancer. I agree with this thinking, and have no complaints. I'm glad to make this small contribution to medical science. It just underlines the fact of life I've noticed repeatedly since my cancer started, that the future is hard to predict.[6]

Dr. Tolcher did tell Gordon that since the study opened no one had stayed in it more than eleven months. It seemed no one could live any longer with unleashed T cells. Gordon found all the information Dr. Tolcher gave him quite tolerable. He was willing to risk the "wasting" and found the one-in-three odds acceptable. His only concern was getting in. Whether he was deemed eligible was ultimately Merck's call. Dr. Tolcher would submit his records to the drug company; it would rule "yea or nay" most probably by the end of the week. Merck would also tell START whether Gordon should receive infusions once every two weeks or once every three weeks. According to Dr. Tolcher, both options were equally favorable; the frequency of treatment did not appear to influence the outcomes.

After a day of tests and appointments, Gordon was in the mood to see some sights. For $1.20 (less than half the fare we pay at home) he caught a bus heading downtown. En route, he was amused to see a fellow passenger who looked like an escapee from one of the many hospitals in the area—a man dressed in a shapeless blue cotton top and baggy pants, grey socks, and no shoes. Gordon wondered what his story was. In the center of town, he walked along car-free walkways beside the San Antonio River. Then sitting outside as the cool air drifted off the water, he drank Lone Star beer, ate barbequed brisket, listened to snatches of mariachi music, and watched the riverboats ferrying tourists up and down.

A few hours later, in Vancouver, I wrote: *August 6, 5 am. Can't sleep.* I was worrying. From what Gordon had told me about his conversation with Dr. Tolcher, I knew that we faced two make-or-break moments. If the scan at twelve weeks showed no improvement, Gordon would likely be taken off the trial. If he responded to the drug, he would be supported by the medication for no longer than eleven months—until July 2014. After that, he was on his own. His body would have to manage without the help of MK-3475. Both prospects alarmed me. *I wish Gordon were here. I'd be less scared.*

When Gordon left San Antonio, he began to think that his participation in the trial was probably a go. Everyone was saying, "See you on Monday." Although he did not have Merck's formal approval, the fact the staff expected him to come back struck him as a sign Merck's consent would come.

On August 9, it was official. Gordon was in! First treatment on August 12. However, as if to warn us that we still couldn't rest easy, our enemy launched another salvo—a new lump emerged on Gordon's right arm near his shoulder. We didn't know for sure it was melanoma, but what else could it be? I told myself that at this point, I should be content with the fact that Gordon was in one of the last two slots of the lambro trial without the chemo arm. This should be a cause for celebration. We had ascended the third hill.

Looking back, I thought about all we had done since June 12 when we learned about the brain tumor, and how, though it often felt we were blundering, stumbling in the dark, we did make some of the right calls. If Gordon had walked down the hall to start whole brain radiation on the day we were in Dr. Kim-Sing's office instead of going home, he would have finished the treatment on July 22. The four-week washout would have taken him to August 19—eleven days past Merck's deadline. I didn't think the drug company would have been so accommodating then and Gordon might have missed the trial. Another piece of serendipity was that when the receptionist at Merck asked me what state I wanted, I said "Texas." Had I asked for another, I might well have drawn blanks—studies for which Gordon didn't qualify. It was true, Gordon did not make Dr. Smiljanic's deadline. We were six weeks over, but considering everything that had happened, we did quite well. Not only was Gordon in systemic treatment, he was in useful systemic treatment.

While Gordon's doctors supported his decision to seek out a trial, they did not actually locate it for him. We were largely on our own in that pursuit, which proved to be time-consuming and frequently frustrating. Although ClinicalTrials.gov is supposed to help people find studies, as Dr. Tolcher said, it has "largely not met the level of good enough. What it will do is spew out a large list. But it doesn't make your life any easier to try to track down those studies. Sometimes nobody answers the phone at the numbers given. The eligibility is such that you don't always know if you fully qualify." According to Dr. Tolcher, a solution might be to develop a "medical concierge service." Instead of looking at a long list of experiments, patients would go to a well-informed intermediary who had "the inside track." Just as a hotel concierge can often get you tickets to a Broadway play or other things you wouldn't know how to get yourself, a medical concierge would be able to find slots in a desirable study. Yet, despite the fact that we had hunted, without being able to consult such an expert, we had achieved what we set out to do.

I had reason to congratulate myself on this accomplishment and I did so—briefly. But mostly I was fretting. Would the immunotherapy work? On which side of the Great Divide—Responder/Non-Responder—would Gordon fall?

14

AN UNEXPECTED MOLECULE

The classical music had a crackly, echoey sound, like an old record being played in a large empty room. Even though I was hearing only a digital recording coming through a phone line, it had a poignant air. And then the music stopped and the voice on the line said something to me in Japanese, which I don't speak. I hoped that if I answered in English the person on the other end in Kyoto would understand me.

"May I speak to Dr. Honjo?" I asked.

"Just a minute," the woman said. I waited a couple of minutes and then I heard another voice:

"Hello."

"Is that Dr. Honjo?"

"This is he."

Tasuku Honjo was the man who made the discovery on which Gordon's treatment—and possibly his life—depended. I felt a little shivery thinking about this. I knew that the story of the drug that Gordon had received was complicated. It played out over two continents and involved several investigators, but it had started in Honjo's lab over twenty years ago. Out of a mixture of gratitude and inquisitiveness, I decided to follow the trail and arranged to call the Japanese scientist. Honjo is a professor in the school of medicine at the University of Kyoto, which has a long tradition of research excellence and is home to ten Nobel laureates.

Honjo told me that in high school, he realized an occupation that afforded some independence would suit him. "I knew I wouldn't be good at working for somebody else. I wanted to be on my own." He considered three careers: diplomat, lawyer, or doctor. "I decided finally to be a doctor. One of the reasons was that my father was a surgeon. It was my family business," he said, laughing.

When Honjo was an undergraduate, he read *The Revolution in Biology*, a book that changed his life. In it, the author, Atsuhiro Shibatani, made a prediction that fascinated Honjo: "The day will soon come when, just like a surgical procedure, DNA abnormalities can be corrected with a pair of tweezers."[1] Honjo decided to become an MD and medical researcher. His postgraduate studies were with Osamu Hayaishi, a medical chemist at the University of Kyoto who had worked in the United States at the National Institutes of Health and cultivated a wide circle of international connections. Hayaishi held noon seminars for his students to which he invited guest speakers from a range of scientific disciplines. "I enjoyed them very much," said Honjo. Like his mentor, Honjo went to the United States for a couple of years; he was a visiting fellow at the Carnegie Institute and the National Institutes of Health. He came back to Japan, took a position at Osaka University, and then in 1984 moved to the University of Kyoto, where he has been ever since.

Though Honjo discovered a molecule that was important for the understanding and control of cancer, he didn't set out to do anything of the sort. The improbable journey began on the day that a graduate student of his, Yasumasa Ishida, came to him with a proposal. He wanted to isolate the gene responsible for T cell selection. The thymus receives juvenile T cells from the red bone marrow and "educates" them so that they become functional—able to destroy invaders or faulty home-grown cells. In the thymus, T cells that attack the body's own healthy cells are induced to apoptosis, or programmed cell death. In less technical terms, you can say they commit suicide. The thymus exerts rigorous quality control; 98 percent of T cells don't make the grade. Ishida wanted to understand the gene involved in this process.

"Originally I didn't agree," said Honjo, "because I was not working on the T cell." Honjo was researching another type of white blood cell, the B cell. (Unlike T cells, B cells cannot kill flawed cells directly; instead, they produce proteins that poison invaders as they travel through the bloodstream.) Ishida was persistent, however. "We had a long discussion," said Honjo, "and eventually I asked him to go ahead." After a couple of years, Ishida discovered a new gene that was expressed when T cells were provoked to apoptosis. It produced a protein on the surface of those cells that did not appear when they died for other reasons. Honjo gave the gene and the protein it made, the ominous-sounding name Programmed Cell Death-1, or PD-1.

Before talking to Honjo, I read an interview with him in which he compared one of the joys of research to picking up an ordinary stone everyone else had disregarded, and discovering, after polishing it for ten or twenty years, that it was a diamond.[2] I asked him whether PD-1 was such a stone. "I think so," he said emphatically. In 1992, when Ishida and Honjo published their paper about PD-1 in *Embo*,[3] a deafening silence greeted the news. Honjo expected that other scientists would be interested in the discovery of the novel gene—that they would request a clone in order to experiment with it themselves. "But we didn't receive any requests. Nobody cared. Nobody tried to duplicate our results."

A few years later, Honjo realized that PD-1 was not in fact needed to induce apoptosis. Though the gene's name turned out to be a misnomer, Honjo decided to keep it anyway. He still believed PD-1 was important because in the experiment Ishida had conducted, it produced high levels of protein, suggesting it fulfilled some critical role. But what? The most straightforward way to discover the function of PD-1 was to inactivate or knock out the gene in mice and observe what happened. If the behavior or physiology of the mice changed, scientists could surmise the gene's function. The method for doing this was new, and "for us it was a challenge," said Honjo. To learn more about the technique, he sent one of his students, Toro Nakano, to Tak Mak, an innovative geneticist in Toronto. When Nakano came back to Japan, he showed another student of Honjo's, Hiroshi Nishimura, how to create knockout mice.

Nishimura set to work. After two years, he was "very much disappointed" with his results, Honjo remembered. The mice that lacked PD-1 "were just fine" at three months. This seemed to indicate that the new gene did not play a significant part after all, and that the time Nishimura spent setting up the experiment was wasted. Fortunately, Nishimura didn't kill all the mice that appeared to be so discouragingly healthy. His patience was rewarded. Once the mice reached between six months to a year of age, they began to develop symptoms of a lupus-like disease in which the immune system causes widespread inflammation and tissue damage. Furthermore, when mice, genetically at risk for other autoimmune diseases such as diabetes, were deprived of PD-1, those diseases started sooner and the effects were more severe. Honjo and Nishimura published the results of the knockout experiment in 1999.[4] PD-1 was definitely an immune system regulator that prevented the body from destroying itself. It was akin to CTLA-4, which Jim Allison had already investigated, although its effects were less dramatic. (Mice deficient in CTLA-4, died within weeks of being born, a powerful demonstration of that gene's vital importance.)

PD-1 was a signaling molecule—like CTLA-4. But how exactly did it work? What messages did it receive? And from where? What signals did it send? Honjo called a biotechnology company in Boston, to see if he could find some answers. This eventually led him to Gordon Freeman, a scientist who played a leading role in the next phase of the story.

When I called Freeman to learn more about how events unfolded, I opened our conversation by asking how he had become interested in science. His absorption, Freeman recounted, began in high school.

> I'm from the far suburbs of Fort Worth, Texas. I grew up a Texan and loved playing football. I don't have a Texas accent because I had a speech defect as a kid and had to take speech therapy. It gives me this fake British accent. I was born in the '50s when Sputnik was a shock to American confidence. The U.S. panicked over our level of scientific expertise and really funded science education all the way down into the high school level and beyond.

Among other things, alarm over the Russian advance boosted the importance of the National Science Foundation, which Harry Truman had established in 1950. In 1956, the year before Sputnik, the foundation received $40 million in government funds, and two years after Sputnik it received more than triple that—$134 million.[5] Flavin Arseneau, a teacher at Freeman's high school, Arlington Heights, used a grant from the foundation to set up a lab that introduced students to the scientific method. "It was inspirational," Freeman recalled. The National Science Foundation also funded summer research programs for high school students at colleges, including one that Freeman attended at the University of Texas in Austin. This was the same program that James Allison had enjoyed, although the two budding scientists did not meet then.

"Jim's a couple of years older than me," Freeman pointed out. He also recalled:

> I was a Texas kid without bigger horizons. I didn't have much vision of applying to college outside of Texas but doing well in this program told me I could play in the big leagues. Somehow I got into Harvard and have stuck around since. I think the program was an investment worth making.[6]

In 1985, Gordon Freeman arrived as a postdoctoral fellow at the Dana Farber Institute, an organization affiliated with Harvard. He started studying B7, an intriguing protein that had both stimulatory and inhibitory effects on the immune system. Then he began to search for other molecules structurally similar to B7. The Human Genome Project was under way, giving investigators like Freeman rich sources of information. "When we started there were maybe two hundred known genes. But when they started sequencing the whole genome, suddenly the databases had little pieces of all sorts of new genes. We went looking for cousins of what we already knew was interesting."

In 2000, Freeman found another promising protein in the B7 family.[7] It happened that his molecule was what Honjo had been hoping to unearth, a molecular mate to his PD-1. Freeman's molecule was its ligand, fitting into the receptor molecule on the T cell like a key in a lock. When the ligand met its "lock," it sent a message—a negative signal that prevented the T cell from proliferating. Freeman dubbed the protein PDL-1 (the L stood for *ligand*). A year later, he detected a second ligand, which he called PDL-2. Freeman emphasized that PD-1 and its ligands were part of the body's routine way of slowing down an immune reaction. PDL-1 was expressed on normal somatic cells to protect them from attack, to prevent autoimmune disease.

> The immune system is hard to get going. You don't want it to start too easily because you might damage too many things. Once you get it started, it's like a two-ton boulder rolling down a hill. You need to slow it and eventually stop the immune response. PDL-1 is one of the natural mechanisms for slowing down and stopping an immune response after you've successfully eliminated a microorganism.

You won't find much PDL-1 in a healthy person, Freeman explained. But when someone is combating an infection and the immune system is aroused, it makes gamma interferon, which in turn increases the expression of PDL-1 and moderates the immune response. As I heard Freeman saying this, I was reminded of the gleam in Allison's eye when he was speaking about his fascination with T cells: "They don't kill you. Why don't they kill you?" he had asked. The question was simple; the answer, more complicated. The immune system is a formidable engine of destruction, but it is constrained. First, the T cells are rigorously selected in the thymus, and those that might attack the body are rejected. Fittingly, when the immune system is moved to action, it starts gingerly. Allison's work showed that before a T cell is activated, two signals are required. The T cell won't go unless a key is put into the ignition switch and the gas pedal is depressed. It has to recognize an antigen—the characteristic bit of protein that heralds a dangerous pathogen or a defective home-grown cell—as well as receive a second positive signal from a molecule called CD28. But the immune system has additional safety features—like a car, it has more than one brake. Allison had discovered one such system—the CTLA-4 checkpoint. PD-1 inhibition was another.

In 2001, Freeman found that PDL-1 was expressed on breast cancer cells. This was a major breakthrough—our "aha!" moment, he said, "discovering cancer cells could turn off the immune response."[8] Two years later, Freeman extended this insight: "We showed PDL-1 expression on many different types of tumor cells."[9] Several cancers, like normal cells, could deflect the immune system and multiply, undisturbed by the T cells. For a hundred years, doctors had been trying to use the immune system to rid the body of tumors. They had wondered why it was so difficult to do. After all, the system was exquisitely sensitive to viruses and bacteria. Cancers had many peculiar mutations that theoretically should have set off alarm bells. What made them so invulnerable? Now with Allison's research and this new understanding of PD-1 and its ligands, pieces of the puzzle were beginning to align. In fact, the immune system did destroy some malignancies. Freeman noted:

> The body has lots of little cancers which the immune system sees and eliminates before there are any medical problems—at the five-cell or

100-cell stage. When a tumor grows, it takes years to get big and become a medical problem. During those years, the tumor learns to evade the immune response. If it didn't, it would be eradicated. The big way it learns to evade the immune response is to express PDL-1. PDL-1 is cancer's shield.

In the past, researchers hadn't realized that cancers survived by mimicking normal cells and protecting themselves the same way they did. I was tempted to call it a devilishly clever maneuver, although I knew better than that. Tumors weren't clever; but they had developed ways of evading the immune system's surveillance.

For Freeman, the goal was never just intellectual understanding. He wanted to help people, and now he might be able to do it. *This could be important*, he thought. *We might have a target for a therapy*. Medarex, the small pharmaceutical company that was already working with James Allison, also saw the potential. If it could block the interaction of PDL-1 with PD-1, it could potentially create a treatment for cancer. In fairly short order, the company developed an antibody. By using a similar antibody made in his lab, Freeman showed it worked in cell cultures. He saw proof of principle—a robust immune reaction.[10] Describing the antibody's effect on PD-1, he said, "It prevents PDL-1 from coming in. Basically it's like putting your hand over the keyhole. It blocks it, but doesn't function as the key." The antibody ensured that the PD-1 brake was off and the T cells were free to go on the attack. I asked Freeman whether he celebrated the milestone. It was too early at that point, he maintained. "We wanted to see how effective and safe it was in people." We are more complicated than petri dishes, and opportunities always exist for things to go wrong.

Clinical trials in human beings were still a few years off. But more corroboration that Freeman was on the right track emerged from some research he undertook with an old friend of his, Rafi Ahmed, an expert in infectious diseases at Emory University in Atlanta. I spoke to Ahmed just after he had returned from a whirlwind trip to England, Spain, and Singapore. Showing no sign of jetlag, he talked with enthusiasm about the investigations that led to the publication of a most influential paper in 2006.

Ahmed grew up in India, did an undergraduate degree in chemistry there, and in 1970 came to the United States, where he began taking courses in microbiology. "I'm not sure why I started studying it," Ahmed said. "That's the honest answer, but once I started studying it I realized I enjoyed it and I was good at it." He entered the PhD program at Harvard (where he worked one floor below Freeman). He graduated in 1981, and in 1984 he moved to the University of California Los Angeles and opened his own lab.

> I got very interested in the topic of immunological memory. That was the beginning of my career. I really was very fascinated by how, when we get a vaccine as a child or get a childhood infection, we are protected for life. Many of our good vaccines give us lifelong immunity. Questions of immunological memory for infections became a passion with me. I wanted to understand how the immune system can remember a pathogen that we encountered thirty or forty or fifty years back. That has shaped what I have done over the last thirty plus years.

Ahmed learned that "the memory T cells you get after an *acute* infection are very functional cells. Upon reexposure to the virus they can expand again, and kill virus-infected cells." But the situation is quite different when a person has a chronic infection like hepatitis B or AIDS. "We discovered that if you have a chronic infection, you don't get functional memory cells." That realization led Ahmed to ask a couple of related and important questions. Were the T cells eliminated during a chronic infection? Or were they still physically there, but ineffective? The distinction, though subtle, was significant. If the T cells were present but inactive, maybe something could be done to restore their vigor. Fortunately, it turned out that the T cells were not killed but exhausted, played out. This was not good, of course, but the situation was far more hopeful than if the T cells were deleted altogether. It might be possible to revive them. The hunt was on.

When Dan Barber, a graduate student in Ahmed's lab, observed that PD-1 is expressed at very high levels on these exhausted cells, "that was another big moment in our science," Ahmed recalled. If PD-1 played a key role in chronic infections as well as in cancer, then perhaps the same remedies would work for both. It was a tempting idea that cried out to be tested. So Ahmed asked himself, "Well, who has some reagents against PD-1?" It turned out that his friend from graduate school days, Gordon Freeman, had some. Ahmed recalled, "It was a wonderful reunion with Gordon, who, in parallel, was working on PD-1. It was a convergence of two research programs and that's what resulted in our combined paper that came out in 2006." They used mice as test subjects, and the result, according to Ahmed, "was a compelling demonstration that T cell exhaustion can be reversed by a PD-1 blockade."

T cell restraint is part of the delicate balance the immune system strikes. When the T cells are confronted with a stubborn chronic disease, either an infection or a cancer, they eventually stop "trying" to beat the illness. Freeman explained, "Say you have hepatitis. You don't want to fight so hard that you totally burn your liver out. That would be fatal. So in some infections if you don't succeed, you sort of settle into an unhappy medium. We now realize cancer is a long fight with the immune system and the T cells become exhausted and get turned off through PD-1." The work on T cell exhaustion also sheds light on why earlier immunotherapies had failed. Though it seemed quite sensible to try to cure cancer by boosting the immune system, there was a catch-22. The Go and Stop signals are intimately linked. Once a T cell recognizes a cancerous cell or group of cells and becomes active, it also sets in motion the protocols that will slow itself down. As Freeman said: "Once cancer gets ahead in the fight, you have a feedback loop. Every time you put your foot on the gas, you're pressing even harder on the brakes."

Ahmed spoke about this work being a convergence of two research programs. It represented another kind of convergence as well. For years, the studies of cancer and of infectious diseases were considered separate fields. The available treatments were very different; oncologists and infectious disease experts had little to say to one another. But now the mental map we have of disease is being redrawn. Diseases of T cell inhibition are a new large territory comprising two formerly independent principalities.

Trials of PD-1 antibodies in people began to take place in both Japan and the United States. In Japan, Ono Pharmaceuticals bought the rights to the Medarex drug called Opdivo (or nivolumab) and then became a partner with Bristol-Myers Squibb to further develop and test it. The application to give the medicine investigational status went to the FDA in June 2006.[11] In 2010, Suzanne Topalian, head of a research group at Johns Hopkins, ran a small study of nivolumab. The results were tantalizingly encouraging. Then in 2012, she led a multicenter study that

changed the course of cancer therapy. Her trial enrolled 296 patients
with advanced melanoma, lung cancer, prostate cancer, renal cell, and
colorectal cancer. Participants with melanoma did best; in almost 30
percent of the individuals, tumors shrank or dissolved altogether. Moreover, the results were durable. After a year of follow-up, two-thirds of
the patients kept their gains.[12]

Meanwhile, Merck, the second horse out of the research gate, produced its version of an anti-PD-1 remedy and in December 2010 applied to have it approved as an investigational drug. Several successful
clinical trials ensued that showed the Merck drug certainly helped
many patients live longer. It seemed to be more effective than ipilimumab, the first of these immunotherapy drugs, and, remarkably, appeared to have fewer side effects. As Freeman put it, this is probably
because PD-1 is a "subtle" regulator of the immune system. To explain
what he meant he pointed to the knock-out mouse studies. "If you make
a mouse that doesn't have CTLA-4, it's born, but then within two
weeks, it dies because it has massive autoimmune proliferation—attack
everywhere. That suggests you want to have CTLA-4 in your body. You
don't want to turn it off forever." On the other hand, "If you knock out
PD-1, the mouse is fine and lives normally for up to a year or more and
then the mouse gets autoimmunity."

It was a long journey for the molecule Honjo and Ishida had first observed in the early 1990s. Honjo, who as well as being a scientist is a
serious golf player with a handicap of 12, certainly scored when he
accepted Ishida's proposal to look for the gene causing programmed
cell death. "I should stress," Honjo said, "that biological science or
medical science usually takes many years. After an initial discovery in a
model system like a mouse, it takes many years for it to be implemented
into a clinical study. You need much luck and I was very lucky, studying
an unexpected molecule."

For my part, I felt lucky that we were in a new era of melanoma
therapies. However, I was still acutely aware that the anti-PD-1 drug
Gordon was slated to receive did not help everyone. Unless the patients
had T cells that recognized the tumor, the medicine wouldn't work. If
the T cells didn't have the enemy in their sights, no amount of PD-1
antibodies would help. In the future, techniques might be developed

that would increase the likelihood of such identification taking place. But as we were still pioneers, we couldn't turn to any established methods for promoting this. We had to rely on the T cells' native ability. Gordon's T cell army recognized millions of different antigens. What were the odds that one of them could detect the particular melanoma mutation that he had? We had no way of knowing this. Once again, we were in the game of wait-and-see.

15

YOU'VE GOT TO BE KIDDING!

Monday, August 12, San Antonio. Today will be my first treatment.
Will it work? A lot hangs on that. When will I know? That's com-
pletely unclear. Well, not completely. I should have a pretty good
idea in 12 weeks. But perhaps sooner.

At START Gordon had a few blood tests, and then another checkup
with Dr. Tolcher. When he mentioned his new lump, Dr. Tolcher said,
"Duly noted," and jotted the information down. Gordon found that
being infused with MK-3475 was much like getting ipilimumab back
home in North Vancouver, although the new treatment took thirty minutes instead of ninety. He lay on a recliner and read while novel antibodies were delivered to his bloodstream. These same molecules had
coursed through the veins of over a hundred people already and so far,
most of the adverse effects reported were "low grade." Afterward, Gordon felt fine—nothing remarkable, nothing to indicate his immune system had been reengineered.

At the airport, waiting to catch an early afternoon return flight, Gordon picked up a local magazine, *Garden and Gun*, in the bookstore. It
happened to be the food issue, so there were articles like "Behind the
Greens: Inspirational Ingredients" and "Candied Sweet Potatoes with
Pecan Bacon Syrup." But between the recipes and the stories about
artisanal purveyors was a piece about varsity athletics, a straight-shooter
team, illustrated with a photo of seven clean-cut students cradling their
firearms—Krieghoffs, Brownings, Perazzis. Gordon thought the juxta-

position astonishing and brought the magazine back as a souvenir—a reminder that, after all, he had been far from home—in *Texas*.

"A clinical trial does not qualify ever," she said. She paused for a moment. And then to emphasize her point, she repeated, "Ever."

I remember seething at the "ever," white hot anger running through me. What I intended to be a dispassionate inquiry had turned into something else. While Gordon was away, I had phoned an officer at the Medical Services Plan of BC to ask whether we could be reimbursed for some of the costs of participating in a study. It seemed like a reasonable request since both our GP and our oncologist had supported the idea of looking for a study south of the border. But the officer who handled "out of country coverage" didn't appear to think so. I suppose I shouldn't have let myself get angry. The policy wasn't her fault.

Nevertheless, I blurted out, "So what would *you* do if your husband was going to die? What if he had run out of treatment options here? What would *you* do?" I didn't tell her the whole saga of Gordon's illness—the many surgeries, the various treatments, and now the six tumors (seven, if you counted the recent one). I just wanted her to think about being in my shoes. Turning a fraction less frosty, she directed me to a form our oncologist could fill out, as well as to supplementary information describing the rules governing financial reimbursement. They were written in bureaucratese, but clear enough: "The appropriate medical specialist making application on behalf of a beneficiary for pre-approval of out of country new or emerging medical services and treatment under this provision must provide documentation of reputable clinical trials beyond Phase III, published in peer reviewed medical literature."[1] Gordon's trial was a phase I. He was not remotely eligible.

Later, to get more clarification, I phoned a manager at the Medical Services Plan of BC. I asked whether being in a U.S. trial was an added obstacle. The manager to whom I spoke said, "The Canadian medical system under the Canada Health Act is looking at the conventional standard of care accepted by Canadian specialists and physicians here. As soon as it doesn't meet that, under the Canada Health Act, you end up with having choices made and past a phase III clinical trial definitely is a requirement under our system, whether or not you get the care here or in the States." The hurdle wasn't the location but the fact that

Gordon was receiving experimental care. The manager was saying that our system had no obligation to provide it.

I remembered Teresa Petrella's remarks in *New Evidence* that I had read earlier. She had written, "The current standard of care for metastatic melanoma in Canada is clinical trials."[2] This was in direct contradiction to the policy of our provincial medical insurance plan. Clinical trials might be the medical standard of care but evidently not yet the legal standard.

The major expense of the infusions that Gordon would receive was the drug itself. Merck was going to cover that. But the other costs, not negligible, fell to the clinical trial participants. Gordon and I could pay, but where did this leave patients who were financially strapped? Didn't the Canada Health Act guarantee universality—that all eligible residents were entitled to the same level of care—and accessibility—that insured persons should not be impeded by financial or other barriers?

Because our provincial medical insurance would not cover Gordon's expenses in Texas, further consequences ensued. Hope Air, a Canadian charity, provides free flights to patients who need to travel for medical care. But it will only do so if the initial medical appointment is covered by a provincial health-care plan.[3] Since Gordon's appointment was not, his flight would not be either. Kathy Barnard suggested we try the Melanoma International Foundation, "an incredible melanoma organization in the U.S." I inquired, and the president, Catherine Poole, e-mailed me back, saying she could offer a single travel grant of $250. I was touched by her willingness to help but decided to leave the money for someone more in need than we were.

Medicine is changing, and for some conditions, studies are the best options available. As Dr. Paul Martin at the Fred Hutchinson Cancer Research Center in Seattle writes, "Advances in treatments and medications continue at a rapid pace and demonstrate the ability to improve health care outcomes through clinical trials. Patients struggling with chronic, debilitating, and life-threatening diseases must have access to all reasonable avenues of possible benefit, including any appropriate clinical trials that are open for enrollment."[4] For over a decade, the United States has recognized the role that clinical trials can play in helping patients recover from serious diseases. On June 7, 2000, then-president Clinton signed an executive order requiring that Medicare reimburse patients for all the routine care costs they incurred as a result of being in clinical studies. A press release about the order stated that because the Clinton administration was promoting biomedical research (it had increased funding for the National Institutes of Health by $7.3 billion, or 73 percent, since 1993), it seemed only logical to remove financial barriers preventing patients from participating in the trials it was funding.[5] Dr. Tolcher said this established a standard: "Medicare sets certain precedents that other insurers usually follow." According to Paul Martin, further improvements occurred in March 2010, with the passage of the Patient Protection and Affordable Care Act (popularly known as Obamacare) although "major obstacles exist."[6] Some patients still find it difficult to access studies, but at least, the U.S. government has started to make it easier for them to take part; in Canada, we lag behind and patients are losing valuable opportunities.

Gordon didn't tell me what was happening right away. But four days after he got back from San Antonio, he couldn't keep the good news to himself any longer.

While we were busy packing, getting ready for a family vacation at our cottage, Gordon said, "I think it's working."

"What? You've got to be kidding!"

"I thought that's what you'd say. That's why I didn't mention it sooner. But yesterday, I noticed the lump on my shoulder shrinking. Seriously, feel it."

I did so—tentatively. "Hmm," I said. And then cautiously, I warned, "Don't say too much!"

"And the pain in my buttock is less," Gordon added.

I was expecting that even if the lambro were successful, it would take awhile. Allison had told me that in early studies, researchers were surprised that immunological therapies might not show results for as long as six months. How could Gordon see an effect in just a few days?

The next night, after we drove north and settled into our place, I lay awake in our small bedroom. While listening to the loons calling back and forth across the lake, I warned myself, *Don't get your hopes up too much.* It was a strange thought to have, because, of course, for almost two years, we had been working toward just such an outcome. Getting my hopes up was really what I wanted!

I was on an emotional see-saw—my mood going up or down in response to what I regarded as positive or negative signals. I reflected about a story I'd heard recently at a dinner party. One of our friends told us about her son, who had developed what his doctors thought was lung cancer. When a tumor turned up in his groin, they suspected something else was wrong. A biopsy revealed melanoma. He'd never had any skin manifestation of the disease at all—no wayward moles, no small subcutaneous lumps like Gordon. Once the oncologists figured out what was going on, it was too late. Our friend's son, who lived on Vancouver Island, saw Dr. Paul Klimo, Dr. Smiljanic's predecessor, in North Vancouver and visited specialists in Edmonton and Los Angeles. No one could do anything. Melanoma is a devious disease, its course unpredictable. *Best to keep that idea firmly in mind,* I told myself.

And then a once-in-a-blue-moon event confirmed the world could deliver unexpected gifts. At the lake, wildlife sightings are one of the great pleasures. We frequently see deer and moose, less often mink, beaver, coyotes, and foxes. On rare occasions we see bears. Although there are cougars in the area, we have never spotted any. But one morning, when Talia was walking down the path to the boathouse, she noticed Charlie, our cat, running hell-bent-for-leather toward the cottage. She thought nothing of it. Charlie is given to dashing about unexpectedly. Then she saw why he was spooked. One of the elusive big cats was in the middle of the path ahead, next to the tent that she and Pat were using. The cougar and Talia looked at each other. *It is massive!* she judged, and also took off for the house. Calmly the cougar sauntered off into the bush.

Gordon wrote:

August 21. The improvements have continued. I'm quite sure it's working. And not only is it working, it's working without any unpleasant side effects at all—not soreness, inflammation, swelling, no diarrhoea, no nothing! It's amazing!

August 25. The lump on Gordon's shoulder is smaller than a lentil. If you didn't know its history, you wouldn't think twice about it. I wish I knew how the lump on his buttock was doing. He thinks it is getting softer and hasn't had to take any more Tylenol for pain. Gordon said, "Now that the melanoma is under control, I can get back to my life." It seems rash to say that. Scary.

August 29. I still have moments of fear.

Me: (Feeling Gordon's shoulder). "That lump is growing larger!"
Gordon: "That's me, that's my bone!"
Me: (after feeling around a bit) "Yeah, okay."
Gordon: "Don't be so pessimistic."

On September 3, Gordon flew to San Antonio for his second treatment. Dr. Tolcher told Gordon he was definitely experiencing a response and said most of his patients (all but three or four) who saw one tumor shrink, found the rest did as well. However, he also said that lambro does not cross the blood-brain barrier—a filtering mechanism in the capillaries that carry blood and oxygen to the brain. While this protects the brain from harmful substances, it creates challenges for physicians attempting to minister to it—to supply helpful remedies. We couldn't count on the therapy to obliterate stray melanoma cells in the brain and so Dr. Tolcher advised regular monitoring with MRIs.

A few days later, Gordon and I were in The Hive, a hip center in downtown Vancouver that provided space for nonprofits, entrepreneurs, creative types, activists, professionals, and techies. Kathy Barnard's foundation, Save Your Skin, had organized a symposium there—an information session for patients and their families. After Kathy welcomed us, Dr. Winson Cheung, an oncologist who recently had taken on more responsibility for melanoma at the BC Cancer Agency, gave a presentation. He cited the number of new cases of the disease in Canada every year (5,500) and worldwide (200,000). He said the incidence was rising (3 to 5 percent annually). He also reported that metastatic melanoma had poor outcomes, a fact that was all too familiar to everyone in the room. *He's not taking into account the new treatments,* I decided. Medical breakthroughs did not instantly filter down from journals and conferences to routine practice. When Dr. Cheung offered to take questions, someone asked whether a Gamma Knife might be coming to Vancouver. He said he didn't know, although he mentioned that some stereotactic radiation was being performed in Vancouver anyway.

Dr. Michael Smylie from the Cross Cancer Institute in Edmonton was next. Gordon and I knew he had considerable expertise with novel antimelanoma agents because we had tried three times to get Gordon into one of the clinical trials he was running! He began by sketching out a bit of history. He said that an early immunotherapy, IL-2, did cure some people, but the percentage of successful cases was small—6 percent of patients. Then he described the action of drugs that inhibit genetic mutations responsible for rapid cell growth—BRAF or MEK. While these medications often produced impressive reductions in tumor burden, the effect usually did not last and the cancer commonly returned. But, he said, we were now in an era of changing paradigms. The newest immunotherapies helped more people, and the benefits often endured. He told us that ipilimumab achieves a lasting response in about 10 to 15 percent of patients. He also talked about MK-3475, and I was reassured to hear that it seemed to work best when patients were given 10 mg (per kilogram of their weight) because this was the dose Gordon was getting. At that level, he said the drug shrank tumors in about 45 to 50 percent of individuals.

The group applauded Dr. Smylie enthusiastically and then we broke for socializing, the aspect of the evening I enjoyed most. We met Shannon Gaudette face-to-face; she was the woman to whom Gordon had spoken on the phone when he developed a brain metastasis. Her example had given us hope and we were encouraged to see that she was still healthy. For the first time, we met Bob and Yvonne Gerard, like us, a North Vancouver couple. Bob was the patient in the couple, and when Yvonne described herself as his case manager, I understood completely what she meant. The Gerards told us that like Gordon, Bob had a nodular melanoma—on his scalp. Fairly rapidly, it metastasized to his brain where four tumors developed. He'd had whole brain radiation at the BC Cancer Agency. Although he felt it dealt with cancers he might have had at the cellular level, at the end, he was still left with the original four tumors. So in August 2013, he had Gamma Knife surgery in Winnipeg. I was heartened to see someone else benefiting from a Gamma Knife treatment. We had struggled so hard to reach a conclusion about the appropriate kind of radiation and were gratified to have our reasoning corroborated. Although the evening had its low notes, Gordon and I left feeling empowered. Just encountering survivors who were obviously doing well had a salubrious effect.

When I talked to Talia on the phone, however, she reminded me we still had reason to remain cautious. "Every time we get a bit hopeful," she said, "there's some awful news." She sounded like me! I knew what she was thinking. Gordon had his lymph nodes removed, then found another lump. As we were just starting to relax after Gordon's ipilimumab treatments, a PET scan revealed six tumors. And when he was accepted into the trial at The Angeles Clinic, a brain metastasis was suddenly discovered. Talia's warning echoed some lines of a poem by Carl Sandburg. I read them many years ago and they have always stayed with me:

> Yes, be happy. It's a good nice
> Way to be.
> But not happy-happy, kid, don't
> Be too doubled-up doggone happy-
> Happy people . . . bust hard . . . they
> Do bust hard . . . when they bust.[7]

And then, adding to my concerns, the U.S. government jumped off the so-called fiscal cliff on October 1. All sorts of government operations—including ones that interested me, clinical trials and airports—were affected. The country had reached its debt ceiling of $16.4 trillion and could no longer meet its obligations. Routine functions were shut down, and eight hundred thousand federal employees were sent home on leave while negotiations to raise the debt ceiling were in progress. Normally, the National Institutes of Health admitted two hundred people into trials every week, but now patients who had already been accepted were put on hold indefinitely until the government was up and running again. I had no idea whether START would have similar trouble. Some news stories also predicted that jobs at air traffic control towers staffed by the Federal Aviation Administration would be slashed. What would this do to Gordon's flights? It would certainly have been easier if Gordon had been able to get into a clinical trial in Canada and avoided the lurching craziness of the American political system!

But Gordon received no phone calls from START telling him to stay home, and U.S.-bound flights out of Vancouver did not seem to be impeded. Despite the looming fiscal crisis, Gordon took off to San Antonio for his fourth treatment. Now that he was starting to respond to it, he wanted to know how likely that reaction was to last. Dr. Tolcher told him that in his experience no one who responded to MK-3475 had relapsed.

Gordon's account of his visit was reassuring. I knew that theoretically, immunotherapy had several advantages over traditional remedies and that should help make its effects long-lasting. The T cell army is extraordinarily flexible, ready to go after pretty much anything that is thrown at it. If a cancer mutates, the T cells can respond to the changes. We are not talking about a one-trick pony here. T cells can also remember what they have been exposed to in the past—even thirty or forty years previously—and can eliminate a type of deviant or dangerous cell more quickly the second time round. I understood and appreciated these beneficial features. But I also considered the fact that MK-3475 had a short track record. What unknown side effects might be in store?

At home on the morning of October 16, Gordon complained of "feeling rocky." He had experienced pain in the night—at the back of his head, low down near his neck.

"It's a brain met," I exclaimed.

"The thought crossed my mind," Gordon said, "but I don't think that's it."

"We should try to get the MRI moved up."

"Let's see how it goes. Don't jump to conclusions."

"But that's what I do!"

"We just have to live with the uncertainty."

"It's hard!"

Gordon felt better the next day and went off to see Rob about the results of another biopsy—of a mass in his parotid gland. We had known about this lump since Gordon had the fateful MRI in The Angeles Clinic. But the lump was a low priority and the wheels of investigation had moved slowly. I was nervous and Gordon, as usual, less so. Nothing was found, just blood and debris. So was there a tumor of some sort that the lambro dispatched? Rob remarked, "God loves you." When Gordon related the anecdote, I thought, *Yeah and we got to Merck.*

Talia continued to be anxious. She booked a holiday to Hawaii for the end of November, but told me she got insurance, "in case something awful happens to Dad." Gordon kept having disturbing symptoms: sinus congestion, nightmares, headaches. I read that headaches, especially early in the day, could be a sign of a brain tumor, although of course, they could be a sign of something else as well. One morning I suggested again moving the MRI up. Gordon resisted.

"Let's have breakfast."

And after breakfast, he said, "Let's see how the day goes. I don't want to fly off half-cocked."

Though I was concerned about a brain malignancy, Gordon pointed out that the trouble could be his old weakness, a tendency to develop sinus infections, exacerbated by the frequent flying and the fact that he was taking an immunotherapy. Maybe, he said, he was suffering from an allergic reaction because his immune system was more active. I didn't know if that made sense. What was signal? What was noise?

On November 4, the date of Gordon's fifth visit to START, he had attained the twelve-week turning point. Merck was going to assess his reaction to the medication. If he wasn't responding he would be taken off the study.

Dr. Tolcher was away for a few days, so a colleague, Dr. Drew Rasco, took the appointment. Gordon handed him the disk from the latest CT scan, done at Lions Gate just a few days before. He explained he had not yet seen the report about the scan, but that the technician had promised to fax it down to START.

Dr. Rasco slipped the disk into his computer, opened the CT file, and looked intently at the black and white image. After a few minutes, he smiled and said, "I'm estimating an 80 percent response rate to the MK-3475. This is based on the cross-sectional area of the visible remains of three tumors, including that large one in your buttock. All of these tumors have changed in appearance. They're ragged at the edges, as if something is eating away at them. But I can't really tell whether there is any live cancer left; I may just be looking at dead cells. What I'm giving you is a *conservative* estimate." He also told Gordon that according to Merck's protocol, he had to have another CT scan in a month to confirm the results.

When Gordon asked about the assessment from Lions Gate, Dr. Rasco gave him those findings as well. To Gordon's surprise, they were considerably less conservative than Dr. Rasco's. According to our radiologist, only a single tumor remained—a small one next to the colon. Moreover, it had decreased in size from 1 cm to 5 or 6 mm. The big cancer in Gordon's right buttock was supposedly gone. "It may have been resected," the radiologist wrote.

Later Gordon and I laughed about the radiologists' supposition— that the tumor may have been removed surgically. I was filled with astonishment at what had transpired—that several cancers could quietly vanish, simply dissolve under the T cell barrage. Gordon had some discomfort, to be sure, a few headaches and congestion, but he experienced no pain at the sites of the melanoma tumors, no swelling, no redness. He had no fever or chills. You might experience more of a reaction when purging your body of an ordinary winter cold or flu than Gordon had when clearing out the melanoma. I thought about friends of ours who'd gone through chemotherapy, about the misery they endured, and how I had always assumed that was the price you paid, if you wanted to live.

Why did Gordon respond so rapidly to MK-3475? Not everyone does. Was it the radiation he had? A synergy is reported to exist between radiation and immunotherapy. But the radiation on Gordon's axilla took place about a year before his first infusion of MK-3475, and the Gamma Knife treatment on his brain was a relatively small dose. Was either a factor? Gordon's melanoma was aggressive. Did that mean his tumors were loaded with antigenic mutagens that easily excited the immune system? Do melanomas like Gordon's have an Achilles' heel? The notion has a certain poetic justice. Is it true? I am only speculating.

November 20, 2013. MRI came in yesterday—all clear!

I relaxed a bit knowing there was no evidence of cancer in Gordon's brain. That night I had two dreams. In the first, I was observing chimpanzees in a large enclosure. A male chimp came over to me and looked penetratingly into my eyes. Then he kissed me, put his lips on my forehead, pressed them down for a few minutes and lifted them off. For a second time, he looked deeply into my eyes with his own large brown ones. I found this profound contact with an evolutionary cousin to be healing. I was pleased and I remember deciding I should tell Gordon what had happened. In the next dream, I was driving a car while asleep. Knowing this was dangerous, I dragged myself out of unconsciousness and took control of the careening vehicle. I brought it to a halt just in front of a barrier of some kind. Had I not done so, I would have crashed.

Gordon thought both dreams were auspicious. In his diary he wrote:

> *I think they were dreams of enlightenment: (1) We are part of nature, with no difference in kind, no boundaries separating us from the rest of the natural world; (2) what we are conscious of, we can begin to control.*

The healing power of the chimp's kiss stayed with me and also the lovely feeling of the penetrating gaze, his eyes so sage and kind. Why was that so soothing?

Over the next couple days, melanoma hit the news channels with both positive and negative stories. Researchers conducting a phase I study of MK-3475 for advanced melanoma disclosed at a conference in Philadelphia that four out of five of the patients were still alive a year after they entered the trial. A Merck official called the results "quite striking."[8] I thought they were too—a far cry from the statistics I had seen shortly after Gordon was diagnosed. But then there was another report—about Nick Auden, a forty-one-year-old Colorado man with melanoma who was not helped by standard treatments and was told he was too sick to qualify for a clinical study of an anti-PD-1 therapy. When I spoke to Dr. Tolcher about this, he said:

> That seems hard and uncaring. We're in a profession that's all about compassion and it's painful to have to tell patients they don't qualify but we have to live within the rules of the entry criteria. I've gone to medical lectures, and investigators have said, "Oh the patients shouldn't have gone on the study, they were really close to hospice, and they suddenly responded." Well, they shouldn't have gone on the study. It puffs you up—you performed a Lazarus effect—but if you take a lot of patients like that, they don't have a chance to respond. They are supposed to have a life expectancy of three months. If they are close to death, there's no way you can turn the immune system on, and have enough time for it to actually work. Doctors by their nature want to help patients. It's the reason they went into being physicians, but at the same time, you have to go by the rules.

The directives ensure the scientific validity of the experiments; medical progress depends on them. But patients are also given experimental drugs outside clinical trials—in compassionate care or extended access programs. So after Nick was denied a spot in a study, he asked Bristol-Myers Squib and Merck if they could provide an anti-PD-1 drug to him through one of these channels. Both companies declined to help. Merck cited difficulties in producing enough of the medicine to supply its trials, and Bristol-Myers Squibb had safety concerns.

Amy Auden, Nick's wife, made a video, *Save Locky's Dad,* in which her son pleaded poignantly for his father's life. Half a million people signed a petition asking the pharmaceutical companies to give Nick access to an anti-PD-1 drug, but the corporations did not yield to the moral pressure. Nick died in his home on November 22, 2013.[9] Hearing about Nick reminded me that the "bad old days" are not altogether behind us and that thorny ethical questions confound us still.

The drug companies maintain they can benefit the most people by getting good therapies approved as quickly as possible. They usually only open up compassionate care or extended access opportunities after they are confident that official endorsement is coming. Gordon got ipilimumab through a compassionate care program, but by then, Health Canada had already given it the green light and Bristol-Myers Squibb was just waiting for the BC Cancer Agency to arrange funding. Giving one person early access might open the floodgates to more people wanting the same treatment. Drug companies are concerned that if patients outside clinical trials do not do well with new drugs, confusion about their benefit can arise. Making the case for the novel medicines could become more difficult and acceptance might slow down. These are not idle worries. In 2014, the FDA stopped Los Angeles–based CytRx, from enrolling more people in a clinical trial of Aldoxorubicin. The company had allowed a patient who was not eligible for a study to receive the cancer therapy through a compassionate care program. When the man died, the FDA halted further participation until it could review the study protocols.[10]

But of course, for someone like Nick Auden, being denied a chance at survival is a cruel blow. To be told that his exclusion is required for the greater good does not make it any easier to bear. Nick couldn't enroll in a clinical trial, and the drugs that might have saved him were not approved, so his doctor couldn't prescribe them. Is there any way out of this heartbreaking catch-22?

Dr. Tolcher doesn't think the guidelines about who gets experimental medicines should be fundamentally changed. "For the time being, until a better system comes along, this is the system that has worked, and worked effectively for us." However, he is convinced the testing process can be made more efficient so that at least new medicines become available more rapidly. One problem is red tape. He said, "There is so much bureaucracy to get studies started in many institutions in the United States—even after the FDA has allowed a drug to go to patients for the first time." START streamlined these procedures and was the first clinic to begin testing MK-3475. Dr. Tolcher recounts, "We ran a phase 1 trial for six months or so before we found the correct dose. The other site that was supposed to join us in that first study, the Mayo, hadn't opened the study. Even though they have a reputation, they are bogged down with bureaucracy."

START found additional efficiencies by improving the way in which trial data is transferred to the sponsor. Dr. Tolcher explained: "We invented some novel software which allows us to move our anonymized research data and put it up on the web in a secure environment so our sponsors can look at it and make decisions very quickly. The approval of MK-3475 [September 2014] vindicated the system." The drug was endorsed in slightly over three years—a record. (By comparison, ipilimumab required twelve years, from 1999 to 2011, to move from the first clinical trial to a license.)[11]

An Arctic air mass traveling south through Canada and the American Great Plains in late November dumped four to six inches of snow on the Texas Panhandle. Authorities in Dallas declared the storm "Ice Force Level 1," which meant they would dispatch thirty sanding trucks to deal with perilous road conditions. On November 24, airlines canceled more than three hundred flights at Dallas-Fort Worth International Airport, about one-third of scheduled departures. However, Gordon's seventh trip to San Antonio was rerouted through Phoenix and he arrived only a little behind schedule.

But not all was well. Dr. Tolcher told Gordon he had high levels of creatinine—a waste product of muscle metabolism. This indicated impaired kidney function. Also Gordon's TSH—thyroid-stimulating hormone—was elevated, a consequence of an underactive thyroid gland. Although Gordon had not lost weight, it seemed the T cells were besetting his own body. It was not exactly the "wasting" we had expected, but close enough to it that Dr. Tolcher decided to stop MK-3475—at least temporarily. Gordon said, "The war is over and the soldiers are on furlough starting bar fights around town." Dr. Tolcher smiled and said, "Yes, that's an apt comparison." He prescribed a steroid, prednisone, to settle down the T cells and synthroid to replace the thyroid hormone Gordon's body was not producing.

Because Gordon had reacted so quickly to the MK-3475, I inferred that his T cells were well primed to set upon the melanoma tumors. Why then were they going after his thyroid? After I reflected about this, I realized that the MK-3475 did not just affect the T cells primed to attack melanoma; the drug was a systemic therapy that influenced all of Gordon's T cells. Perhaps some of them had been primed erroneously to attack his thyroid. So long as these T cells were held in check, the thyroid was protected from "friendly fire." But when MK-3475 released the T cells, the thyroid was collateral damage.

Once Gordon got home, on Dr. Tolcher's recommendation he scheduled a combination CT/PET scan. The CT scan was necessary to satisfy Merck's protocol that called for a sixteen-week scan. The PET scan would reveal whether any live cancers remained in Gordon's body—a matter of considerable interest to Gordon and his care team. If he was clear, everyone would feel more comfortable about stopping the treatments. Gordon booked the scan with a private clinic in order to meet Merck's deadline. He was hoping the drug company would pay for it. (Eventually it did, reimbursing us for both the CT and the PET.)

On December 6, with the temperature outside our home hovering slightly below the freezing mark, Gordon drove over to Burnaby for the combination scan.

> *December 11. No PET scan result yet. Should be soon. Gordon feels good—sings in the morning. I like that.*

> *Dec. 12. No PET scan results today. Maybe tomorrow or Monday.*

> *Dec. 13, Friday the 13th. PET scan all clear—astounding! Report says, "In keeping with complete metabolic response to therapy!" Wow!*

So much for ancient superstitions about bad luck on Friday the 13th.

We didn't pop the champagne corks. We were experiencing a walking-on-eggshells kind of happiness—a little guarded. But I did tell our friends that Christmas came early that year and I got the best present ever.

Lambrolizumab was approved by the FDA nine months later. The code name, MK-3475, was more or less dropped and the drug acquired two new monikers instead. The U.S. Adopted Names Council, which looks after such matters, changed its generic name to pembrolizumab, and Merck picked Keytruda as the marketing, or brand, name.[12] In a recent "face-off" trial with ipilimumab, its results were significantly better, and Tony Ribas, an oncologist who worked on early immunotherapy trials, said, "I've been treating melanoma for 15 years. This is the first time I have seen patients with durable responses, and the majority with no side effects. We saw no nausea, no vomiting, while the immune system is attacking the cancer. There is no better personalized therapy than this."[13]

16

NOW, THERE ARE ALL OF YOU

Gordon was intrigued by all the highways and byways of the human soul. In the winter of 2013, his interest began to include a remarkable condition in which people have an intense desire to amputate a healthy arm or leg. "How *could* any sane person want to be rid of a perfectly good limb, which serves them well in all the business of life?" Gordon wrote.[1] Individuals with the disorder reported feeling that a part of their body did not belong to them. Gordon wanted to understand this sense of belonging and not-belonging. Were the individuals afflicted by amputation desire experiencing a converse of the phantom limb phenomenon in which people complained of pains in a limb that did not exist? What could these folks teach us about how we construct our sense of self? Do we have a "body-model" and a "me-model" that might or might not coincide? Gordon finished a long post discussing these perplexing matters in mid-January and then we left for a celebratory trip.

We flew to San Antonio first, where Gordon was scheduled to have a checkup. On our first morning there, the sky was an intense blue. Intermittent gusts caused the trees to sway and ruffled the surface of the San Antonio River. I guessed that the wind blew a lot in the city; the place where we were staying, Inn on the Riverwalk, displayed a sign, "100% powered by wind." I was not expecting to find Green initiatives like this in Texas.

We toured the Alamo, the site of the famous battle in which the Mexicans routed the Texans in March of 1836. A month later, retaliation followed this humiliating defeat. Led by Sam Houston, the Texans beat the Mexicans at the battle of San Jacinto—where the rallying cry was "Remember the Alamo." I will always remember the Alamo too, although what I associate with it will be rather different.

The START clinic was at the northern outskirts of San Antonio—in a district teeming with hospitals, clinics, and research institutions. We drove there on Fredericksburg Road, past strip malls, countless fast food outlets, big-box stores, and crazy blow-up cacti advertising car dealerships. START itself was in a sleek, spacious building befitting its mandate of discovering the latest in cancer therapy. I accompanied Gordon to his appointment, met Dr. Tolcher, and snapped a picture of the two of them beaming at the camera.

After a few days in Texas, we left for New Orleans. I had always loved the music and had wanted to visit the Big Easy for many years. I took to the quirkiness of the city immediately. As we were looking for a place to have dinner on the night we arrived, we noticed that a local realtor, Finis Shellnut, was advertising "Haunted and Not-Haunted apartments for lease." We saw voodoo artifacts for sale—in Rev. Zombie's House of Voodoo—and in antique stores we found objects that spoke of forsaken splendor—chandeliers as big as a small car and silver chafing dishes large enough to contain a whole turkey.

From our hotel, Inn on Ursulines, we tramped all over the French Quarter. We walked to the St. Louis Cemetery No. 1, on the north side of Basin Street, immortalized in "Basin Street Blues" — "Basin Street is the street/Where the best folks always meet/In New Orleans, land of dreams. . . ." We strolled over to Bourbon Street, somewhat tawdry now, and Gordon caught the raunchy venues illuminated by a kaleidoscope of neon lights on film. We checked out a newer music scene on Frenchmen Street, described as "Bourbon Street for the locals." Sitting in a small club, on either side of a small table, we talked and talked about all manner of things, as we always have. Toward the end of the evening, as we left to go to our hotel, we encountered a group energetically jamming in the road. The members had driven up, parked their cars, brought out horns and trombones and begun to play. It was like a climactic scene in a Broadway musical where people suddenly burst into song and instruments appear out of nowhere.

New Orleanians are fond of wrapping you up in their stories. Near Bourbon Street, a young man hailed us, introduced himself as Chris, and asked if we wanted to see his courtyard. Not many visitors to New Orleans get to see something like it, he told us. "Okay," we said. He unlocked a weather-beaten door and we were suddenly inside a still, secluded space filled with tropical plants. Chris was a workman, helping the owner restore and renovate the building by creating a series of suites opening on to the garden. He said, "Come, I'll show you the attic." We trudged up an outside staircase and entered an apartment. Chris pulled aside a panel and pointed. "The secret room," he said confidingly. He told us there were other hidden passageways through-out the building. In fact, it was common in many of the houses in the French Quarter. "Why?" I asked. Chris explained that it all dated back to the days of slavery. The white masters didn't want to see their slaves; they wanted them to keep out of sight as they moved around the own-ers' homes. I was startled by what Chris was telling us—an ugly remin-der of the past.

And then, drinking coffee and eating almond croissants in the Com-munity Café on Royal Street, we heard a more positive story from a man at the next table. Dick Deluxe was a musician who'd knocked about quite a bit. He told us about his gigs, including a few in Vancou-ver (in a famous nightclub called The Cave, which had fake stalactites growing down from the ceiling). Then he mentioned writing a song about Sputnik Munroe, a famous white wrestler from Kansas who started his career in 1945. When segregation was customary at public events, the celebrated fighter wouldn't perform unless blacks were al-lowed to sit anywhere around the ring. I noticed that Dick had a couple of his CDs on the table with him. I couldn't resist buying one, and when we got home and cracked open the case I realized that it contained his song about the folk hero. "Say what you will about Sputnik Monroe/He took a big bite out of old Jim Crow. . . ."

Life in the French Quarter has a congenial, unscripted quality. The looseness reminded me of the jazz for which the city is so famous. I found it stimulating, and I envisaged a new book, in which I could weave together my thoughts on melanoma and medical history. It would bring in ethics and, throughout, there would be the threads of love and affection I have for Gordon, the man who has been my best friend and constant companion for over forty years. Perhaps it is not surprising that here on the Mississippi Delta such thoughts should arise. Many authors have found inspiration here. Tennessee Williams wrote that he could hear that "rattle trap streetcar named Desire running along Royal and the one named Cemeteries running along Canal, and it seemed the perfect metaphor for the human condition."

Back in North Vancouver, Gordon was being monitored for melanoma. His scans were clear, but he still had to take thyroid supplements to compensate for the effects of his treatment. I started reflecting about everything that had happened over the past two years and what it meant. Although Gordon was not receiving infusions any longer, I was struck by the fact that we were still part of the melanoma community. Ten years ago, no community like this existed. Survivors of metastatic melanoma were so rare.

Many individuals contributed to the historic change. Scientists— James Allison, Tasuku Honjo, and others—were clearly key. Impelled by a deep curiosity about how we defend ourselves from disease, they made discoveries about the complex signaling systems that govern T cells. As a result, drug companies developed medications that operated according to new principles. Decades ago, patients with metastatic melanoma usually died despite their doctors' best efforts. Nevertheless, some oncologists were convinced we could do better and were willing to offer new therapies. Patients contributed too, by being willing to try them. Sometimes the chance these novel medicines would help was remote, but they gave it a go, thinking that at least the knowledge gained might help others.

Among those early pioneers was Kathy Barnard who did not accept that she had only six months to live and who carried on. In so doing, she illuminated the way for the rest of us. "I don't want to be the last man standing. It's a guilty place to be," she said. Kathy has supported many melanoma patients in their journeys—both emotionally and practically, helping them to find useful medicines and connect with knowledgeable physicians.

Like Kathy, Bob Gerard got a similarly grim verdict, but he and his wife, Yvonne, kept searching for a cure nonetheless. Gordon and I first met the Gerards at a Save Your Skin symposium in September 2013 and we got together several times after that. Over coffee one morning at the Gerards' house, Bob told me he had noticed something on his scalp late in the summer of 2012 but didn't do anything about it for several months. He explained, "I always had this ingrained belief that I was never going to get cancer. It was so powerful in me. I was going to have a healthy life. I was going to live a full life. I was immune to it all."

After Yvonne urged Bob to have the lesion checked, he eventually saw a dermatologist who excised the lump in early December 2012. Two days after the procedure, he received a devastating report. It described an advanced nodular melanoma—large, aggressive, and ulcerated. Scans in January and February 2013 were clear. Nevertheless, Bob was uneasy. He felt light-headed all the time—as though he had just drunk a couple of glasses of wine. The sensation was not in itself disagreeable, but he thought it indicated something was wrong. His sense of being immune to trouble had vanished and he kept prodding his doctors for a diagnosis. In May, his GP gave him the results of a full-body CT scan: "I'm afraid I have bad news. . . ." Afterward, when Bob picked Yvonne up from work, he said, "It's in my brain." Yvonne suddenly felt cold—ice cold.

Five days later, Yvonne and Bob were both in a morning meeting at the BC Cancer Agency to discuss radiation. Yvonne had taken eight weeks' compassionate leave from work—granted in BC to employees with a family member who is "gravely ill." She didn't like having to acknowledge how serious Bob's condition was, but taking the time off made it easier for her to help him. In the meeting, the Gerards learned that Bob's situation was perilous; he needed whole brain radiation—immediately. He had four tumors, so surgery was out of the question. "There was no discussion of any options," said Bob. He had his first treatment right away; nine more sessions completed the regimen. The day of the last one, another shock: Bob read a summary of his treatment and discovered it was described as "palliative." He knew he was in trouble, but he hadn't realized quite how much.

The whole brain radiation stopped the tumors from growing. Bob also felt it probably dealt with any micrometastases he might have had. But it didn't destroy the four original tumors. They were a lurking menace. Bob and Yvonne wondered if further therapy might be appropriate. Yvonne started making phone calls about clinical trials. By then, the Gerards had met Kathy Barnard, who suggested they contact Dr. Smylie in Edmonton. "A second opinion is never a bad idea," she counseled. Bob and Yvonne flew to see Dr. Smylie in July. "Our conversation with him was simple," Bob recalled. "I'd recommend that your next step be stereotactic radiation," he said.

After the Gerards returned home, Bob had a couple of conversations with a radiologist at the BC Cancer Agency about stereotactic radiation. A significant hitch emerged. Bob had four tumors, and the local equipment could handle three at most. He couldn't be treated in Vancouver. Fortunately, the Gerards were already prepared for this eventuality. They had done some research and learned about Gamma Knife surgery, which could remove a half dozen or more tumors. They made inquiries at two Canadian facilities that offered it—in Toronto and Winnipeg. The center in Winnipeg had opened its doors in 2003 and was the first in Canada to provide Gamma Knife. Dr. Derek Fewer, a neurosurgeon at the Winnipeg clinic, was also the first to respond to the Gerards. He assured them that Bob was a good candidate for the technique. When they asked who would pay for the procedure, he said, "Just get here, and we will make the funding arrangements." Since Gamma Knife surgery was necessary, approved in Canada, but not available in BC, our BC provincial insurance picked up the tab. The local radiologist they had been consulting wrote a letter to explain that he could not provide what Bob needed. Bob was treated in Winnipeg on August 8. His tumors began to disappear and now he has only one left, but it too is shrinking. So far, it has gone down from 1.2 cm to 4 mm.

I was surprised to learn that radiation might take so long to shrink a tumor, but apparently this is not unusual. The American Cancer Society reports: "Radiation doesn't always kill cancer cells or normal cells right away. It might take days or even weeks of treatment for cells to start dying, and they may keep dying off for months after treatment ends. Tissues that grow quickly, such as skin, bone marrow, and the lining of the intestines are often affected right away. In contrast, nerve, breast, brain, and bone tissue show later effects."[2] Bob and Yvonne recently celebrated the second-year anniversary of Bob's radiosurgery. They went out to dinner and drank a glass of bubbly. "It was a very memorable day for us," Bob said.

In December 2014, I attended another Save Your Skin gathering. Patients and their spouses were invited to have lunch, and the survivors could have their stories recorded. I remember Kathy Barnard beaming at the gathering of people and saying, "I used to be the only one, and now, there are all of you." I got goosebumps as I listened to her and looked around the room at the smiling faces.

During that Save Your Skin event, I met another man with a remarkable story. Nigel Deacon, a retired school principal and university teacher, lives in Victoria. In June of 2010, he was diagnosed with ocular melanoma—a rare disease affecting about five in one million people. Though these tumors in the eye can be eradicated with radiation, some of them are at high risk for metastasizing to the liver. Once this happens, the chances of survival are markedly reduced. (The Ocular Melanoma Foundation still reports on its website, "There are no approved treatments for OM [ocular melanoma] once it has spread.")[3] Despite the sobering prognosis, Nigel was not afraid. "I just got on with my life." He continued to teach part-time at UBC.

Early in 2012, Nigel went to India where he spent several months in intense yoga practice. On his return home in March, he developed an excruciating pain in his abdomen. Imaging showed a large mass between his liver and his pancreas. A subsequent scan showed that the tumor was growing and creating satellite malignancies. "There were two tumors in my liver. It was really looking awful," Nigel recalled. An oncologist in Victoria offered him dacarbazine. Nigel turned down the suggestion, "because it just makes you sick and is completely ineffective." He told his oncologist, "I need to look for other things."

At the beginning of the summer, he went to see a second oncologist in Vancouver to discuss the possibility of a treatment (other than dacarbazine). The doctor was not encouraging. In many places, patients with metastatic ocular melanoma had not been able to participate in the immunotherapy "revolution." They had been excluded from clinical trials of ipilimumab because they had such poor outcomes in general and the new immunotherapy was expected to be no better.[4] However, Nigel kept investigating his condition on the Internet and became convinced there were, in fact, viable options. In August, he drew up a selection of possible therapies and went to see the oncologist in Vancouver again. Nigel said, "In the United States people are trying these things. Some people are having success and I want to try too." At that point, the physician had an idea: "There is a person in North Vancouver who may be able to get you ipilimumab on a compassionate basis."

The person in North Vancouver was Dr. Sasha Smiljanic, who did indeed get Nigel ipilimumab through Bristol-Myers Squibb's compassionate care program. Nigel had four infusions in the fall of 2012. But in January 2013, scans showed that despite the medicine, the tumors were becoming larger and multiplying.

By then, Nigel had a new oncologist in Victoria, Dr. Vanessa Bernstein. She said, "You're not responding. It's time to register with a hospice." Later she explained to me on the phone that because Nigel's scans were not good, and there were not a lot of treatment options left, she thought it was wise to prepare. "But I didn't think he was about to die immediately." Nigel put his name on the list; nevertheless, he hadn't given up. He remembered, "There was another part of me that said, 'This can't be true. I cannot accept this.'"

Nigel had radiation in March and April to shrink some of his tumors and his condition stabilized. He also set himself a challenge. If he could succeed, he thought, "Then I will know that I will not die in the near future." Nigel was a runner, and for years had heard about a race called the Comrades Marathon in South Africa. It was an ultramarathon, quite a test, even for someone who had not registered with a hospice. The route would take him along 87 kilometers from Durban to Pietermaritzburg, up in the mountains of KwaZulu-Natal, 825 meters above sea level. Nigel told me, "I knew that if I could survive, if I could get to the top of those mountains, then I would know the story was not over. My body would not be able to do that if I was really dying." What he called "Nigel's impossible dream" came true. Not only did he complete the marathon, but in the process, he raised money for African children with HIV/AIDS. "That set me on a track," Nigel said. "Everything became possible again even if not probable."

By reading more about ocular melanoma on the Internet, Nigel gathered that Dr. Takimi Sato in Philadelphia was one of North America's foremost experts in the disease. In the fall of 2013, he went to visit him. "He's like a saint to us," Nigel said. Because ocular melanoma is such a rare cancer, Nigel thought that only a few people would actually garner the experience with it that he needed. Nigel told me that when Dr. Sato examined his latest scans, his view was surprisingly optimistic. He said, "It looks to me like you're not finished yet. I don't think this cancer is running madly inside your body." Dr. Sato told Nigel that he was getting a mixed response, there were some new tumors, but some were getting smaller, and some had stopped growing. Nigel was experiencing a delayed reaction to ipilimumab; this was not unusual in response to an immunotherapy. As Nigel recalled, Dr. Sato concluded by saying, "That's okay; that fits with the picture, you are responding. And although you have a cancer in your liver and it's really dangerous, it's mostly outside the liver. I'm recommending that you try ipi a second time."

Nigel got a letter from Dr. Sato outlining his encouraging assessment, and when he returned home he showed it to Dr. Bernstein.

"Do you think you could get ipi?" Nigel asked her. By now the BC Cancer Agency was funding the drug. However, as Dr. Bernstein explained to me, "the use of ipilimumab for melanoma was in its infancy at the BCCA at that time and asking to retreat patients was still very new. Ipilimumab costs $100,000 for four doses. So while we could get approval for one course of therapy for a patient, whether we were going to get approval for a second course of therapy really was on a case-per-case basis." Dr. Bernstein was not sure that she would receive authorization, but she sent off an application citing some published data on the efficacy of retreatment with ipilimumab.

The next day, she phoned Nigel. She had a welcome surprise: "It's been approved."

Nigel had his second round of ipilimumab and finished before Christmas 2013. He said, "In January 2014, we were looking at quite a different picture. Some tumors had disappeared."

The tide was beginning to turn for ocular melanoma and ipilimumab, not just for Nigel but for other patients as well. In May 2013, a small ground-breaking European study had found that 31 percent of patients with ocular melanoma were alive one year after ipilimumab treatment.[5] By October 2013, the BCCA had decided to offer the innovative therapy to patients with ocular melanoma.[6]

When I last spoke to Nigel in August 2015, he said, "There are still some active tumors in my body, but they are less active and they are only active on the surface. All of the tumors have died inside. They show up looking quite funny on the PET/CT scans." Nigel has had no further treatment since the second round of ipilimumab. His oncologist continues to monitor him, but so far he is doing remarkably well. The average survival time after a diagnosis of metastatic ocular melanoma is seven months. It has now been more than three years past his diagnosis. If the remaining tumors don't dissolve, Nigel is considering a clinical trial, perhaps at The Angeles Clinic with Dr. Omid Hamid. The hospice in Victoria keeps phoning him to see when he will be coming in, but that date is receding into the indefinite future. Nigel said, "I seem to be falling into thinking of myself as a normal person and not in any more danger than anybody else who walks the streets and gets on buses and things. There's danger everywhere. We don't worry about it."

One lesson you can draw from these stories is "Don't give up"—or, perhaps more accurately, "Don't give up too easily," because, of course, there is always some point at which it makes sense to call it quits. I remember that Rob once said, "I tell patients, 'Never give up, unless you're sitting on death's door. You just never know.'" A corollary: do your own investigations. Not surprisingly, perhaps, it takes a while for everyone to catch up to the new reality. The U.S. FDA gave ipilimumab the green light in March 2011, but Tim Turnham, executive director of the Melanoma Research Foundation, whom I interviewed in 2014, pointed out that not all oncologists adopted it immediately. "Interestingly in the United States about a fourth of melanoma patients last year were treated with dacarbazine. I think it's the lack of penetration, lack of awareness, and some cancer doctors not staying on top of the field. It's not right, it's not good care." More confirmation of the slow "penetration" of ipilimumab comes from the National Comprehensive Cancer Network's survey of over five hundred physicians in May 2013; 56 percent were not prescribing ipilimumab as a first-line therapy for metastatic melanoma.[7]

Nigel credits his own diligence with helping him to find an appropriate treatment. He recognizes that not everyone can do what he did. "Because I'm able to do research and I have a university education, I have a real advantage. But some people are older or sicker. It's just not imaginable that they would try to fight off this terrible enemy." For patients like this, groups like Save Your Skin or the Melanoma Research Foundation can play an important role. Turnham agrees: "One of the things we are looking at very seriously is how we can help, how we can be a voice for more patients. What do we do about those patients who don't tend to go to the Internet and look for treatment options, who don't have access to the good treatment centers?"

Melanoma is as capricious as ever. Usually the primary cancer materializes somewhere on the skin, but in 5 to 10 percent of cases, it develops inside the body, in the lymph nodes or internal organs. Some forms, such as the nodular type that Gordon had, continue to be misdi-

agnosed. *The New Zealand Medical Journal* recently reported that nodular melanomas are missed 50 percent of the time as "they often have
no distinctive clinical features."[8] The disease can spread rapidly after its
initial appearance, but it may lie in wait for several years before causing
serious trouble. In Gordon's case, half a dozen metastases were scat-
tered throughout his abdomen and torso before one arose in his brain.
With Bob Gerard, the cancer jumped directly from his scalp to his
brain, and never emerged in the rest of his body at all. Melanoma is a
dangerous, mutating shape-shifter. But our therapies are getting better
and the melanoma community keeps expanding.

The drugs that have helped to combat melanoma are now being
tried on other cancers as well—of the lung, kidney, and prostate. Early
trials look promising, and oncologists will probably use immunotherapy
widely in the years to some—an important resource for them, to add to
the surgery, radiation, and chemotherapy already in their toolkits.

In this book, I emphasized what we can do for ourselves when a deadly
and difficult disease strikes. I wrote about people who did their own
research, sought out second opinions, and if necessary, traveled to find
the help they needed. Bob Gerard went to Edmonton and Winnipeg,
Nigel Deacon consulted a doctor in Philadelphia, and Gordon visited
clinics in Seattle, Santa Monica, and San Antonio. In order to think
effectively about his condition, and to help him relay his history to new
doctors, Gordon kept his own binder of medical records and a list of his
various procedures and the dates they had occurred. In this era, when
laypeople are beginning to take more responsibility for their health
care, some in the medical world argue that we should do away with the
word *patient* altogether. Julia Neuberger is one of them:

> The word "patient" conjures up a vision of quiet suffering, of some-
> one lying patiently in a bed waiting for the doctor to come by and
> give of his or her skill, and of an unequal relationship between the
> user of healthcare services and the provider. The user is described
> simply as suffering, while the healthcare professional has a title, be it
> nurse or doctor, physiotherapist or phlebotomist.
>
> Patient comes from the Latin "patiens," from "patior," to suffer or
> bear. The patient, in this language, is truly passive—bearing whatev-
> er suffering is necessary and tolerating patiently the interventions of
> the outside expert. The active patient is a contradiction in terms, and

it is the assumption underlying the passivity that is the most dangerous. It is that the user of services will remain passive in sickness,
allowing the healthcare professional to take the active part and tell
the user what to do. The passive patient will do what he or she is told,
and will then wait patiently to recover. The healthcare professional is
the healer, while the recipient of healthcare services is the healed,
and does not need to take a part in any decision making or in any
thinking about alternatives.

If we are to see greater participation in their own care by users of
services, and greater public awareness of what can and cannot be
done, then the term user, despite its lack of elegance, at least con-
jures up an active role. It could even suggest an equalisation of status
between health professional and service user that is nearer the cli-
mate in which modern health services should be provided. The active patient is a contradiction in terms, but the confident service
user, informed and participative, is someone one might hope to see
in most healthcare settings.[9]

I did not adopt this proposal about mothballing the word *patient*, in
part because Neuberger's alternative, *user*, and others such as *client*,
consumer, and *customer* don't seem to quite capture important aspects
of the relationship between physicians and the persons they are caring
for either. Physicians have obligations that other providers of goods and
services don't have. Patients are often vulnerable and afraid, and in
need of compassion as much as expertise. Nevertheless, I endorse the
idea that patients should take an active role in the search for a cure.
After all, they are in a unique position to discover and report symptoms.
Bob Gerard noticed a subtle but important sign—light-headedness. By
urging his doctors to pay attention to it, he probably sped up the treatment of his brain tumors. For Gordon, participating in a clinical trial
was a key part of getting to a cure, but finding that trial was a protracted
affair. Since his harried doctors couldn't undertake such a search themselves, we embarked on it.

However, being persistent and proactive is not the whole story. Patients who survive metastatic melanoma are also lucky. Factors outside
their control fall the right way. They have the right genes—or their
tumors do—so that they can benefit from therapies that are available. I
know that Gordon's determination could only go so far. Melanoma still

overtakes active, resourceful patients. They should not be regarded as remiss; the enterprise is chancy, after all.

When, in March 2012, standing in our front hall I wondered rather dolefully, "What is going to happen to us now?" I certainly did not envisage the tumultuous years that followed. My mother, who alarmed us by breaking her hip during the same week that we learned about Gordon's metastasizing melanoma, is ninety-five now. She still lives in her own home with a caregiver. She often tells us she had a good life. My son, Tom, suffered from symptoms of post-concussion syndrome for over two years. We were aware that when the concussive effects last that long they are very likely to be chronic. But our concerns abated when Tom announced that he was returning to university. He is working on a PhD in economics and is deep into the analysis of Turkish tweets. My daughter, Talia, left publishing and also went back to university to pursue a second degree—in computer science. She is happily writing Apple apps. Our cat, Charlie, still hunts rats. Recently he upped the ante by leaping through an open window into our bedroom, and releasing a live one under the bed. I buried myself under the covers leaving Gordon to deal with "the situation." He picked up the rat by the tail and dropped it out the window.

Gordon's scans continue to be clear of melanoma, but he did not get off scot-free. His thyroid did not recover and he continues to take daily supplements. Mysteriously, he became dissatisfied with his writing about the Phantom Self. The development was completely unexpected, because while we were struggling with the melanoma, those ideas nourished him:

> My diagnosis of melanoma last year did not keep me awake nights. As one gloomy event after another unfolded, my anxiety levels remained low. Claudia worried more than I did; and I worried more on her behalf than on my own. Death is not a problem so much for the one who dies as for the survivors. I can't prove it, but I think my views about persons—about what we are—helped my peace of mind. [10]

Neither of us knows why it happened, but Gordon's book is now in abeyance. I hope that he will return to the project. As he also wrote:

Our lives are strange hybrids of what we strive for and what happens to us. We charge ahead on the path we carve out for ourselves, until something stops or diverts us. We never have as much control as we want; we operate in ignorance of facts that can make or break our most important projects; yet we are far from helpless. We experiment as we go, and sometimes find new ways to push back our limitations.[11]

Gordon did invite his "long-lost" cousin, Linda, and her family to our cottage on Sheridan Lake, and they came for a whirlwind five days. We weren't able to kayak in the summers of 2012 and 2013, due to Gordon's treatments, but in 2014, we explored the Deer Group Islands, famous for their sea caves, in Barkley Sound. In 2015, together with Tom and Talia, we circumnavigated Vargas Island in Clayoquot Sound. We camped on the west coast of the island, at Ahous Bay, a part of the traditional lands of the Ahousaht people, and on the north coast, on a beach abutting Calmus Passage. One rainy day, under a tarpaulin shelter, Gordon baked cinnamon buns in our Outback oven. We shared them with a German family of kayakers who had taken a day trip and come back to the campsite completely drenched. They were surprised and delighted. Generosity is a tradition on these trips; we have often been the beneficiaries. I remember once being given sockeye salmon that was barbequed in a rack of cedar strips over burning embers.

When the rain stopped and the clouds lifted I could see across to Flores Island, the scene of many of our previous adventures. I thought back to the day in June two years before when I was sitting in our kitchen on our old blue stool, head in my hands, thinking that because of Gordon's brain metastasis, we wouldn't be together much longer. But here we were again, and the future was stretching out a little bit ahead of us. We did not know what it contained, but, for the moment, the idea of having a future was enough.

NOTES

INTRODUCTION

1. "Mellifluous," https://www.google.com/search?q=mellifluous&ie=utf-8&oe=utf-8, accessed September 17, 2015.

2. Keiran Smalley, "A Brief History of Melanoma. From Mummies to Mutations," *Melanoma Research* 22, no. 2 (April 2012): 114–22, doi: 10.1097/CMR.0b013e328351fa4d.

3. Ibid.

4. S. Woolhandler et al., "Costs of Health Care Administration in the United States and Canada," *New England Journal of Medicine* 349 (August 21, 2003): 768–75.

5. M. B. Lens and M. Dawes, "Global Perspectives of Contemporary Epidemiological Trends of Cutaneous Malignant Melanoma," *The British Journal of Dermatology* 150, no. 2 (2004).

6. Demytra Mitsis et al., "Trends in Demographics, Incidence, and Survival in Children, Adolescents and Young Adults (AYA) with Melanoma: A Surveillance, Epidemiology and End Results (SEER) Population-based Analysis," *Journal of Clinical Oncology* 33, no.15 supplement 9058 (May 20, 2015).

7. "Crowdsourcing," Merriam-Webster.com, 2011, http://www.merriam-webster.com, accessed September 24, 2015.

I. A PIMPLE-LIKE THING

1. The class was Shotaro Iida's Introduction to Buddhism.

2. Gordon Cornwall, "Introduction," *The Phantom Self,* accessed September 18, 2015, http://phantomself.org/introduction.

3. Married people who develop cancer are less likely to have a metastasizing malignancy and to die of their disease than unmarried people. This suggests the illness is usually discovered earlier, when it is easier to treat. Paul Nguyen et al., "Marital Status and Survival in Patients with Cancer," *American Journal of Clinical Oncology,* September 23, 2013, doi: 10.1200/JCO.2013.49.6489.

4. "Brief Information on Nodular Melanoma," Victoria Melanoma Service, accessed September 23, 2015, http://www.alfredhealth.org.au/Assets/Files/265_Brief_information_on_nodular_melanomas-text_only.pdf.

2. WHAT'S REAL AND WHAT ISN'T?

1. Peter McGee, *Kayak Routes of the Pacific Northwest Coast: From Northern Oregon to British Columbia's North Coast* (Vancouver: Greystone Books, 2004), 204.

2. Claudia Cornwall, "Map of Shame," *Reader's Digest*, September 2010, 72–79.

3. Steven Wang, *Beating Melanoma: A Five-Step Survival Guide* (Baltimore: The Johns Hopkins University Press, 2011), 15.

4. Richard Wooster et al., "Mutations of the *BRAF* Gene in Human Cancer," *Nature* 417 (June 27, 2002): 949–54, doi: 10.1038/nature00766.

4. THE MAD RUSH

1. Steven Wang, *Beating Melanoma: A Five-Step Survival Guide* (Baltimore: The Johns Hopkins University Press, 2011), xi.

2. Vito W. Rebecca, Vernon K. Sondak, and Keiran S. M. Smalley, "A Brief History of Melanoma: From Mummies to Mutations," *Melanoma Research* (April 22, 2012): 114–22, doi: 10.1097/CMR.0b013e328351fa4d.

3. By 1981, researchers had shown that if chemotherapy were added to surgery, 77 percent of patients survived five years without relapsing. With surgery alone, only 45 percent of patients did. Gianni Bonadonna and Pinuccia Valagussa, "Dose-Response Effect of Adjuvant Chemotherapy in Breast Cancer," *New England Journal of Medicine* 304 (January 1, 1981): 10–15, doi: 10.1056/NEJM198101013040103.

4.   The BC Cancer Agency was still not checking for the BRAF mutation. However, in an information bulletin, the agency explained that if patients had metastatic melanoma, the drug company, Roche, would provide the test. Individuals who were positive for the mutation were eligible for Roche's Zelboraf. The BC Cancer Agency agreed to fund Zelboraf from mid-August 2012 onward. Until then, Roche committed to making the medicine available through a compassionate care program. Roche also agreed to supply the BRAF test to prospective patients up to the end of December 2012. "Systemic Cancer Therapy," *The BC Cancer Agency* 15, no. 10 (October 2012), accessed October 4, 2015, http://www.bccancer.bc.ca/systemic-therapy-site/Documents/Update-Oct2012_Supplement10Oct2012.pdf.

5.   Health Canada approved ipilimumab in February 2012, and the BC Cancer Agency began to consider whether it would pay for the drug. Until the funding came through, Bristol-Myers Squibb pledged to provide it in a compassionate care program from June 2012 onward. "Systemic Cancer Therapy," *The BC Cancer Agency* 15, no. 6 (June 2012), accessed October 17, 2015, http://www.bccancer.bc.ca/systemic-therapy-site/Documents/Update-Jun2012_01Jun2012.pdf.

6.   A recent study of how cancer patients use the Internet states: "Survey after survey shows that although patients desperately wish to communicate by e-mail with physicians, in the United States only 6% to 9% of patients have done so." Gunther Eysenbach, "The Impact of the Internet on Cancer Outcomes," *A Cancer Journal for Clinicians* 53, no. 6 (November/December 2003): 356–71. The patients may be on to something; another study found that e-mail communication improves outcomes: Yi Yvonne Zhou, Michael H. Kanter, Jian J. Wang, and Terhilda Garrido, "Improved Quality at Kaiser Permanente through E-Mail between Physicians and Patients," *Health Affairs* 29 (July 2010): 1370–75, doi: 10.1377/hlthaff.2010.0048.

5. DON'T WORRY ABOUT IT

1.   Jeffrey S. Weber et al., "Extended Dose Ipilimumab with a Peptide Vaccine: Immune Correlates Associated with Clinical Benefit in Patients with Resected High-Risk Stage IIIc/IV Melanoma," *Clinical Cancer Research* 17, no. 4 (February 15, 2011): 896–906, doi: 10.1158/1078-0432.CCR-10-246.

2.   Emily Jackson, "Toronto Man Dies without Access to Bristol-Myers Squibb Experimental Drug," *The Toronto Star*, July 11, 2012.

3.   Michael A. Postow et al., "Immunologic Correlates of the Abscopal Effect in a Patient with Melanoma," *New England Journal of Medicine* 366 (March 8, 2012): 925–31, doi: 10.1056/NEJMoa1112824.

4. E. Bastiaannet, J. Beukema, and H. Hoekstra, "Radiation Therapy Following Lymph Node Dissection in Melanoma Patients: Treatment, Outcome and Complications," *Cancer Treatment Reviews* 31, no. 1 (February 2005): 18–26, doi: 10.1016/j.ctrv.2004.09.005.

5. S. Agrawal, J. M. Kane, B. A. Guadagnolo, et al., "The Benefits of Adjuvant Radiation Therapy after Therapeutic Lymphadenectomy for Clinically Advanced, High-Risk, Lymph Node-Metastatic Melanoma," *Cancer* 115, no. 24 (December 15, 2009): 5836–44. doi: 10.1002/cncr.24627.

6. Gordon Cornwall, "The Fog of Medicine," *The Phantom Self*, August 2, 2012, accessed September 23, 2015, http://phantomself.org/melanoma-journal-2/2-aug-2012-the-fog-of-medicine/.

7. Carl von Clausewitz, "On the Theory of War," in *On War,* accessed September 23, 2015, http://www.gutenberg.org/files/1946/1946-h/1946-h.htm.

8. Benjamin Djulbegovic, "Lifting the Fog of Uncertainty from the Practice of Medicine," *British Medical Journal* 329, no.7480 (December 18, 2004): 1419–20, doi : 10.1136/bmj.329.7480.1419.

9. The requirements have changed since 2012. "Health Canada approves Yervoy (Ipilimumab) for first-line treatment of adults with metastatic melanoma, the most deadly form of skin cancer," September 16, 2014, Bristol-Myers Squibb Canada, http://www.bmscanada.ca/en/news/releases, accessed September 17, 2015.

10. Cornwall "The Fog of Medicine."

11. Ibid.

12. Ibid.

13. Ibid.

14. Ibid.

15. Canada suffers from a shortage of PET scans. The World Health Organization recommends countries have two publically funded clinical scanners per million people. Canada only has 0.86 per million. (The United States has 6.5.) Susan Martinuk, *The Use of Positron Emission Tomography (PET) for Cancer Care Across Canada*, AAPS, Inc. and Triumf, 2011, 13.

16. During an online interview about "haggling down" your health care costs, Jen Wieczner, a reporter for the *Wall Street Journal* and *MarketWatch*, said, "In a situation where the bill is $2,000, you might be able to get the price to $500 if you're willing to pay cash upfront." Lizzie O'Leary, "How to Negotiate Your Health Care Bills," *Marketplace,* September 13, 2013, accessed September 23, 2015, http://www.marketplace.org/topics/your-money/health-care/how-negotiate-your-health-care-bills. My search on Google using the terms *negotiating health care costs in the U.S.* netted 2,280,000 results. The topic clearly has traction.

17. Cornwall, "The Fog of Medicine."

18. M.B. Lens and M. Dawes, "Global Perspectives of Contemporary Epidemiological Trends of Cutaneous Malignant Melanoma," *The British Journal of Dermatology*, 150, no.2 (2004).

19. Teresa Petrella et al. "Canadian Perspective on the Clinical Management of Metastatic Melanoma," *New Evidence, Oncology Issue*, September 2012.

20. Ibid.

21. Reshma Jagsi et al., "Real-Time Rationing of Scarce Resources: The Northeast Proton Therapy Center Experience," *Journal of Clinical Oncology* 22, no. 11 (June 1, 2004): 2246–50, doi : 10.1200/JCO.2004.10.083 JCO.

22. Cornwall, "The Fog of Medicine."

23. Letter dated July 04, 2012, from BC Cancer Agency files, Vancouver Cancer Centre.

24. Wang, *Beating Melanoma*, xi.

25. Cornwall, "The Fog of Medicine."

26. Ibid.

6. WE HAVE NO WAY OF
MONITORING SUCCESS

1. Julia V. Burnier and Miguel N. Burnier, eds., *Experimental and Clinical Metastasis: A Comprehensive Review*, New York: Springer, 2013, 301.

2. Significant immune-related adverse events were generally reversible and appeared to be associated with improved relapse-free survival. Weber et al., "Extended Dose Ipilimumab with a Peptide Vaccine."

3. Wang, *Beating Melanoma*, 47.

7. THE ICONOCLAST: A VISIT WITH
JAMES ALLISON

1. "Search for a Cure," *Newsweek*, December 16, 1985, 60.

2. Martin's political career came to an inglorious end when he enlisted a cousin to shoot at him in the summer of 1981. Claiming to be the victim of a satanic cult, he thought he might garner sympathy that would help him in a bid for the Texas Senate. He was, however, charged with perjury. After he fled, the police found him inside a stereo cabinet and apprehended him. He resigned his seat. Paul Burka, Kaye Northcott, and Victoria Loe, "The Ten Best and the Ten Worst Legislators," *The Texas Monthly*, July 1981, accessed September

24, 2015, http://www.texasmonthly.com/story/ten-best-and-ten-worst-legislators/page/0/7.

3. Pierre Golstein, "A New Member of the Immunoglobulin Superfamily—CTLA-4," *Nature,* 328 (July 16, 1987): 267–70, doi: 10.1038/328267a0.

4. Elke Jäger and Alexander Knuth, "The Discovery of Cancer/Testis Antigens by Autologous Typing with T Cell Clones and the Evolution of Cancer Vaccines," *Cancer Immunity* 12, no.6 (May 1, 2012).

5. Cailin Moira Wilke, Shuang Wei, Lin Wang, Ilona Kryczek, Jingyuan Fang, Guobin Wang, and Weiping Zou, "T Cell and Antigen-Presenting Cell Subsets in the Tumor Microenvironment," in T. J. Curiel, ed., *Cancer Immunotherapy*, New York: Springer, 2013, 17, doi: OI 10.1007/978-1-4614-4732-0_2.

6. Dana Leach, Matthew Krummel, and James Allison, "Enhancement of Antitumor Immunity by CTLA-4 Blockade," *Science* 272 (March 22, 1996): 1734–36.

7. G.Q. Phan, J. C. Yang, R. Sherry, et al., "Cancer Regression and Autoimmunity Induced by Cytotoxic T Lymphocyte-Associated Antigen 4 Blockade in Patients with Metastatic Melanoma," *Proceedings of the National Academy of Sciences of the United States of America* 100, no. 14 (July 8, 2003): 8372–77, doi:10.1073/pnas.1533209100.

8. Ibid.

9. Drew M. Pardoll, "Immunology Beats Cancer: A Blueprint for Successful Translation," *Nature Immunology* 13, no. 12 (December 2012).

10. Elisabeth Rosenthal, "When Drug Trials Go Horribly Wrong," *The New York Times*, April 7, 2006.

11. Mae-Wan Ho and Joe Cummins, "London Drug Trial Catastrophe—Collapse of Science and Ethics," *Institute of Science in Society*, July 4, 2006, accessed September 23, 2015, http://www.i-sis.org.uk/LDTC.php.

12. "Ipilumumab," *Wikipedia,* accessed September 23, 2015, http://en.wikipedia.org/wiki/Ipilimumab.

13. "Pfizer Announces Discontinuation of Phase III Clinical Trial for Patients with Advanced Melanoma," New York, April 1, 2008, accessed September 23, 2015, http://press.pfizer.com/press-release/pfizer-announces-discontinuation-phase-iii-clinical-trial-patients-advanced-melanoma.

14. L. A. Jones and M. L. Salgaller, "Immunologic Approaches to Antigen Discovery for Cancer Vaccines," *Expert Opinion on Investigational Drugs* 9, no. 3 (March 2000): 481–90.

15. F. Stephen Hodi, Steven J. O'Day, and David F. McDermott, "Improved Survival with Ipilimumab in Patients with Metastatic Melanoma," *New England Journal of Medicine* 363 (August 19, 2010): 711–23, doi: 10.1056/NEJMoa1003466.

8. A CLOUD OF UNCERTAINTY

1. Sheryl M. Ness, "Cancer Survivors Struggle with Fear of Frequent Scans," February 16, 2013, Mayo Clinic, accessed September 23, 2015, http://www.mayoclinic.org/diseases-conditions/cancer/expert-blog/cancer-and-scans/bgp-20056419.

2. C. A. Thompson et al., "Surveillance CT Scans Are a Source of Anxiety and Fear of Recurrence in Long-Term Lymphoma Survivors," *Annals of Oncology* 21, no. 11 (April 27, 2010): 2262–66, doi: 10.1093/annonc/mdq215.

3. Sasha Smiljanic, "Oncology Notes," May 5, 2013.

9. A HAIRY WEEK SO FAR

1. Antoni Ribas, Caroline Robert, Adil Daud, et al., "Clinical Efficacy and Safety of Lambrolizumab (MK-3475, Anti-PD-1 Monoclonal Antibody) in Patients with Advanced Melanoma," *Journal of Clinical Oncology* 31 (2013) suppl; abstr 9009.

2. "Merck Announces Breakthrough Therapy Designation for Lambrolizumab an Investigational Antibody Therapy for Advanced Melanoma," White house Station, New Jersey, April 24, 2013, accessed September 23, 2015, http://www.mercknewsroom.com/press-release/research and development news/merck-announces-breakthrough-therapy-designation-lambrol.

3. ClinicalTrials.gov lists over thirty-six thousand sites that are recruiting. Of those 41 percent are in the United States, 53 percent are outside the United States, and 6 percent are in the United States and outside it as well. The fact that so many non-American researchers choose to register their studies on ClinicalTrials.gov means that it is a valuable source of information for patients all around the world. ClinicalTrials.gov., accessed September 17, 2015, https://clinicaltrials.gov/.

4. In October 2013, the World Medical Association signed an accord in Helsinki that enshrined the idea that all participants in a clinical study deserve to gain from positive knowledge acquired. Principle 34 of the agreement states: "In advance of a clinical trial, sponsors, researchers and host country governments should make provisions for post-trial access for all participants who still need an intervention identified as beneficial in the trial." "World Medical Association, Declaration of Helsinki—Ethical Principles for Medical Research Involving Human Subjects," 64th WMA General Assembly, Fortaleza, Brazil, October 2013.

10. IT'S NOT BRAIN SURGERY

1.   Dante Alighieri, "The Inferno," trans. John Ciardi (New York: Random House, 1996).

2.   Gordon Cornwall, "It's Not Brain Surgery (Well, Actually It Is)," *The Phantom Self* (June 27, 2013), accessed September 23, 2015, http://phantomself.org/melanoma-journal-2/7-27-june-2013-its-not-brain-surgery-well-actually-it-is/.

3.   Ibid.

4.   Ibid.

5.   This restriction may be undergoing a reevaluation. Historically, patients with brain metastases from melanoma had a poor prognosis because of concerns that drugs would not penetrate the blood-brain barrier. A recent article argues that because patients with brain metastases are surviving longer and some new therapies are able to attack brain cancer, "a reassessment of absolute exclusion of brain metastasis patients from clinical trial eligibility is warranted." But any such reassessment would take several years to come into effect, not soon enough for Gordon. See Jaclyn C. Flanigan, Lucia B. Jilaveanu, Mark Faries, et al., "Melanoma Brain Metastases: Is It Time to Reassess the Bias?" *Current Problems in Cancer* 35, no. 4 (July–August, 2011): 200–10.

11. THE FIRST HILL

1.   Atul Gawande, "Letting Go," *New Yorker*, August 2, 2010.

2.   Ibid.

3.   Ibid.

4.   "Gamma Knife Surgery," *Neurological Surgery in Winnipeg*, accessed September 23, 2015, http://www.wrha.mb.ca/prog/surgery/gamma_knife/.

12. BECAUSE I AM AN OPTIMIST

1.   Emory McTyre, Jacob Scott, and Prakash Chinnaiyan, "Whole Brain Radiotherapy for Brain Metastasis," *Surgical Neurology International* 4, Suppl 4 (May 2, 2013): S236–S244, doi : 10.4103/2152-7806.111301.

2.   Roy A. Patchell et al., "A Randomized Trial of Surgery in the Treatment of Single Metastases to the Brain," *New England Journal of Medicine* 322 (February 22, 1990): 494–500, doi : 10.1056/NEJM199002223220802.

3. Gordon Cornwall, "The Second Hill," *The Phantom Self*, July 12, 2013, accessed September 23, 2015, http://phantomself.org/melanoma-journal-2/8-12-july-2013-the-second-hill/.

4. Abigail L. Stockham and Nils D. Arvold, "The Role of Radiation in the Management of Brain Metastases," *OncLive,* March 6, 2014.

5. Steven W. Hwang et al., "Adjuvant Gamma Knife Radiosurgery Following Surgical Resection of Brain Metastases: A 9-Year Retrospective Cohort Study," *Journal of Neuro-Oncology* 98, no. 1 (May 2010): 77–82.

6. Nick Mulcahy, "'Critical Step': Drug Slows Cognitive Loss after Radiation," Medscape Medical News, November 1, 2012, accessed September 24, 2015, http://www.medscape.com/viewarticle/773768.

7. This is corroborated by several papers, including this one: Mohammad K. Khan, Niloufer Khan, Alex Almasan, et al., "Future of Radiation Therapy for Malignant Melanoma in an Era of Newer, More Effective Biological Agents,"*OncoTargets and Therapy 4* (August 9, 2011): 137–48, doi: 10.2147/OTT.S20257.

8. David Raben et al., "Stereotactic Body Radiation Therapy for Melanoma and Renal Cell Carcinoma: Impact of Single Fraction Equivalent Dose on Local Control," *Radiation Oncology* 6, no. 34 (April 2011), doi:10.1186/1748-717X-6-34.

9. Roy Patchell found that 18 percent of patients who had a single brain metastasis removed surgically followed by radiotherapy relapsed; among those patients who did not have the radiation follow-up, 70 percent relapsed. Roy A. Patchell et al., " Postoperative Radiotherapy in the Treatment of Single Metastases to the Brain: A Randomized Trial," *Journal of the American Medical Association* 280, no. 17 (November 4, 1998).

10. Cornwall, "The Second Hill."

11. Ibid.

12. Ibid.

13. Ibid.

13. WE HAVE TWO SLOTS LEFT

1. In October 2013, the World Medical Association would sign an accord in Helsinki governing the ethical conduct of clinical trials. One of the principles stated that investigational drugs should be compared to the *best* of standard interventions. Perhaps at the time Dr. Hamid's trial was designed, dacarbazine was the best standard therapy available. Subsequent lambro trials would probably use ipilimumab—not dacarbazine—in the control group.

2. "Anti–PD-1 Antibody Produces Durable, Ongoing Response in Patients with Advanced Melanoma," *The ASCO Post,* June 2, 2013.

3. "Immunity Let Loose," *Nature* 498 (June 13, 2013): 140–41, doi: 10.1038/498140d.

4. "Antibody Wakes Up T-cells to Make Cancer Vanish," *The New Scientist,* June 4, 2013.

5. Liz Szabo, "New Drugs Brighten Outlook for Melanoma," *USA Today,* May 29, 2013.

6. Gordon Cornwall, "The Experiment," *The Phantom Self*, September 2013, accessed September 2015, http://phantomself.org/melanoma-journal-2/9-16-sep-2013-the-experiment/.

14. AN UNEXPECTED MOLECULE

1. "The Fruits of Curiosity and Courage in Research," *Kyoto University Research Activities* 4, no. 4 (March 2015).

2. Ibid.

3. Yasumasa Ishida, Yasutoshi Agata, Tasuku Honjo, et al., "Induced Expression of PD-1, a Novel Member of the Immunoglobulin Gene Superfamily, upon Programmed Cell Death," *EMBO Journal* (November 11, 1992): 3887–95.

4. H. Nishimura, M. Nose, and T. Honjo, "Development of Lupus-like Autoimmune Diseases by Disruption of the PD-1 Gene Encoding an ITIM Motif-Carrying Immunoreceptor," *Immunity* 2 (August 11, 1999): 141–51, doi: http://dx.doi.org/10.1016/S1074-7613(00)80089-8.

5. "The National Science Foundation: A Brief History," accessed September 21, 2015, http://www.nsf.gov/about/history/nsf50/nsf8816.jsp.

6. Gordon Freeman and James Allison, both alumni of the summer program at the University of Texas at Austin, made discoveries that contributed to the development of three drugs—nivolizumab, lambrolizumab, and ipilimumab. Sales of those medicines are expected to reach nearly $5 billion annually. "Ipilimumab—FDA's Top 10 Blockbuster Decisions," *Fierce Biotech*, accessed September 21, 2015, http://www.fiercebiotech.com/special-reports/fdas-top-10-blockbuster-decisions/ipilimumab-fdas-top-10-blockbuster-decisions; Arlene Weintraub, "Merck's Melanoma 'Game-Changer' Keytruda Likely to Bolster Drug Pricing Debate," *FiercePharma*, September 5, 2014, accessed September 21, 2015, http://www.fiercepharma.com/story/mercks-melanoma-game-changer-keytruda-likely-bolster-drug-pricing-debate/2014-09-05; Lynne Taylor, "B-MS Mivolumab to Dominate NSCLC Drug Market by 2022," *Pharma Times* (July 15, 2013), accessed September 21, 2015, http://www.

pharmatimes.com/Article/13-07-15/B-MS_nivolumab_to_dominate_NSCLC_
drug_market_by_2022.aspx.

7. G. J. Freeman, A. J. Long, T. Honjo, et al., "Engagement of the PD-1
Immunoinhibitory Receptor by a Novel B7 Family Member Leads to Negative
Regulation of Lymphocyte Activation," *The Journal of Experimental Medicine*
192, no. 7 (October 2, 2000): 1027–34, doi: 10.1084/jem.192.7.1027 .

8. Y. Latchman, C. R. Wood, T. Chernova, et al., "PD-L2 Is a Second
Ligand for PD-1 and Inhibits T Cell Activation," *Nature Immunology* 3 (March
2, 2001): 261–68, PMID: 11224527.

9. Julia A. Brown, David M. Dorfman, Gordon J. Freeman, et al., "Block-
ade of Programmed Death-1 Ligands on Dendritic Cells Enhances T Cell
Activation and Cytokine Production," *The Journal of Immunology* 170 no. 3
(February 1, 2003) 1257–66. doi: 10.4049/jimmunol.170.3.1257.

10. Ibid.

11. Bristol-Myers Squibb Company Briefing Document for the Pediatric
Subcommittee of the Oncologic Drugs Advisory Committee Meeting November 5, 2013, 5, accessed September 24, 2015, http://www.fda.gov/downloads/
AdvisoryCommittees/CommitteesMeetingMaterials/Drugs/OncologicDrug-
sAdvisoryCommittee/UCM373173.pdf.

12. Suzanne L. Topalian, F. Stephen Hodi, Julie R. Brahmer, et al.,"Safety,
Activity, and Immune Correlates of Anti–PD-1 Antibody in Cancer," *New
England Journal of Medicine* 366 (June 28, 2012): 2443–54, doi: 10.1056/NEJ-
Moa1200690.

15. YOU'VE GOT TO BE KIDDING!

1. "Medical Services Commission Out of Province and Out of Country
Medical Care Guidelines," January 19, 2011, http://www2.gov.bc.ca/gov/
DownloadAsset?assetId=5E56E19772E649E493501CCE3A40CE32&
filename=ooc_funding_guidelines.pdf.

2. Teresa Petrella et al., "Canadian Perspective on the Clinical Management of Metastatic Melanoma."

3. "Eligibility Criteria for Free Flights to Non-Emergency Medical Appointments," *Hope Air*, accessed September 22, 2015, http://www.hopeair.ca/
FeaturePage.aspx?pgid=6&mst=~/wwd/WhatWeDo.master.

4. Paul J. Martin, " Responsibility for Costs Associated with Clinical
Trials," *Journal of Clinical Oncology* 32, no. 30 (October 20, 2014): 3357–59,
doi : 10.1200/JCO.2014.57.1422 JCO.

5. "President Clinton Takes New Action to Encourage Participation in Clinical Trials," June 7, 2000, accessed June 17, 2015, http://archive.hhs.gov/news/press/2000pres/20000607.html.

6. Martin, " Responsibility for Costs Associated with Clinical Trials."

7. Carl Sandburg, "Snatch of Sliphorn Jazz," *Harvest Poems* (New York: Harcourt, Brace & World, Inc., 1960) 86.

8. Nick Mulcahy, "Survival 81% at 1 Year with MK-3475 in Melanoma," *Medscape*, November 21, 2013, accessed September 24, 2015, http://www.medscape.com/viewarticle/814825.

9. Sydney Lupkin, "Dad Pleading for Unapproved Cancer Drug Dies," *Good Morning America*, November 25, 2013.

10. Alexander Gaffney, "Company's Compassion Leads to Clinical Hold on Experimental Drug," *Regulatory Affairs Professional Society*, November 19, 2014, accessed September 21, 2015, http://raps.org/Regulatory-Focus/News/2014/11/19/20780/Companys-Compassion-Leads-to-Clinical-Hold-on-Experimental-Drug/

11. The fact that ipilimumab, or Yervoy, was first in a class of new drugs may have increased the length of time the clinical trials took. Drugs that are licensed by the FDA normally go through 6–7 years of testing in phase 1 to phase 3 clinical studies. For the FDA to assess the evidence and grant the license can take up to 2 years longer. "The Drug Development and Approval Process," FDAReview.org, accessed September 17, 2015, http://www.fdareview.org/approval_process.shtml.

12. For more about the business of naming drugs, see Eva Vivean, "Overview of Generic Drugs and Drug Naming," *Merck Manual*, accessed September 21, 2015, https://www.merckmanuals.com/home/drugs/brand-name-and-generic-drugs/overview-of-generic-drugs-and-drug-naming.

13. Alice Goodman, "Practice-Changing Study: Pembrolizumab Outperforms Ipilimumab in Advanced Melanoma," *The ASCO Post* 6, no.8 (May 10, 2015).

16. NOW, THERE ARE ALL OF YOU

1. Gordon Cornwall, "Amputation Desire (BIID/Xenomelia) and the Human Experience of Self," *The Phantom Self*, accessed September 24, 2015, http://phantomself.org/amputation-desire-biidxenomelia-and-the-human-experience-of-self/.

2. "Radiation Therapy Principles," American Cancer Society, accessed October 9, 2015, http://www.cancer.org/treatment/treatmentsandsideeffects/

treatmenttypes/radiation/radiationtherapyprinciples/radiation-therapy-princi-ples-how-does-radiation-work.

3.   "Treatment of Metastatic Disease," Ocular Melanoma Foundation, accessed October 2, 2015, http://www.ocularmelanoma.org/metstreatment.htm.

4.   M. Maio, R. Danielli, V. Chiarion-Sileni, et al., "Efficacy and Safety of Ipilimumab in Patients with Pre-treated, Uveal Melanoma," *Annals of Oncology* 24: 2911–15, no. 11 (2013), doi:10.1093/annonc/mdt376.

5.   Ibid.

6.   "BCCA Protocol Summary for the Treatment of Unresectable or Metastatic Melanoma Using Ipilimumab," accessed October 20, 2015, http://www.bccancer.bc.ca/chemotherapy-protocols-site/Documents/Melanoma/US-MAVIPI_Protocol_1Oct2013.pdf.

7.   "NCCN Trends," *National Comprehensive Cancer Network* (May 2013), accessed September 17, 2015, https://www.nccn.org/store/Products/Trends/pdf/Summary/NCCN_Trends_Metastatic_Melanoma_2013-05-01_Summary.pdf.

8.   Amanda Oakley, Marius Rademaker, and Mark Elwood, "Missed Melanomas—Comment," *New Zealand Medical Journal* 127, no. 1398 (July 8, 2014).

9.   At the time Neuberger wrote this, she was CEO of the King's Fund in London, England, a charity that shapes health care policy. Now she is a Liberal Democrat member of the British House of Lords. Julia Neuberger, "Do We Need a New Word for Patients?" *British Medical Journal* 318, no. 7200 (June 26, 1999): 1756–58.

10.   Cornwall, "The Experiment."

11.   Ibid.

BIBLIOGRAPHY

Agrawal, S., Kane, J. M., Guadagnolo, B. A., et al. "The Benefits of Adjuvant Radiation Therapy after Therapeutic Lymphadenectomy for Clinically Advanced, High-Risk, Lymph Node-Metastatic Melanoma." *Cancer* 115, no. 24 (December 15, 2009): 5836–44. doi: 10.1002/cncr.24627. http://www.ncbi.nlm.nih.gov/pubmed/19701906.

"Antibody Wakes Up T-cells to Make Cancer Vanish." *The New Scientist*, June 4, 2013.

"Anti–PD-1 Antibody Produces Durable, Ongoing Response in Patients with Advanced Melanoma." *The ASCO Post* (June 2, 2013).

Bastiaannet, E., Beukema, J., and Hoekstra, H. "Radiation Therapy Following Lymph Node Dissection in Melanoma Patients: Treatment, Outcome and Complications." *Cancer Treament Reviews* 31, no.1 (February 2005): 18–26. doi: 10.1016/j.ctrv.2004.09.005.

"BCCA Protocol Summary for the Treatment of Unresectable or Metastatic Melanoma Using Ipilimumab." Accessed October 20, 2015. http://www.bccancer.bc.ca/chemotherapy-protocols-site/Documents/Melanoma/USMAVIPI_Protocol_1Oct2013.pdf.

Bonadonna, Gianni, and Valagussa, Pinuccia. "Dose-Response Effect of Adjuvant Chemotherapy in Breast Cancer." *New England Journal of Medicine* 304 (January 1, 1981): 10–15. doi : 10.1056/NEJM198101013040103.

"Brief Information on Nodular Melanoma." The Victoria Melanoma Service. Accessed September 23, 2015. http://www.alfredhealth.org.au/Assets/Files/265_Brief_information_on_nodular_melanomas-text_only.pdf.

"Briefing Document for the Pediatric Subcommittee of the Oncologic Drugs Advisory Committee Meeting." Bristol-Myers Squibb Company. November 5, 2013. Accessed September 24, 2015. http://www.fda.gov/downloads/AdvisoryCommittees/CommitteesMeetingMaterials/Drugs/OncologicDrugsAdvisoryCommittee/UCM373173.pdf.

Brown, Julia A., Dorfman, David M., Freeman, Gordon J., et al. "Blockade of Programmed Death-1 Ligands on Dendritic Cells Enhances T Cell Activation and Cytokine Production." *The Journal of Immunology* 170, no. 3 (February 1, 2003): 1257–66. doi: 10.4049/jimmunol.170.3.1257.

Burka, Paul, Northcott, Kaye, and Loe, Victoria. "The Ten Best and the Ten Worst Legislators." *The Texas Monthly* (July 1981). Accessed September 24, 2015. http://www.texasmonthly.com/story/ten-best-and-ten-worst-legislators/page/0/7.

Burnier, Julia V., and Burnier, Miguel N., eds. *Experimental and Clinical Metastasis: A Comprehensive Review.* New York: Springer, 2013.

ClinicalTrials.gov. Accessed September 17, 2015. https://clinicaltrials.gov/.

Cornwall, Claudia. "Map of Shame." *Reader's Digest.* September 2010.

Cornwall, Gordon. "Amputation Desire (BIID/Xenomelia) and the Human Experience of Self." *The Phantom Self* (January 18, 2014). Accessed September 18, 2015. http://phantomself.org/amputation-desire-biidxenomelia-and-the-human-experience-of-self/.

———. "Introduction." *The Phantom Self* (July 14, 2009). Accessed September 17, 2015. http://phantomself.org/introduction/.

———. "It's Not Brain Surgery (Well, Actually It Is)." *The Phantom Self* (June 27, 2013). Accessed September 23, 2015. http://phantomself.org/melanoma-journal-2/7-27-june-2013-its-not-brain-surgery-well-actually-it-is/.

———. "The Experiment." *The Phantom Self* (September 2013). Accessed September 2015. http://phantomself.org/melanoma-journal-2/9-16-sep-2013-the-experiment/.

———. "The Fog of Medicine." *The Phantom Self* (August 2, 2012). Accessed September 23, 2015. http://phantomself.org/melanoma-journal-2/2-aug-2012-the-fog-of-medicine/.

———. "The Second Hill." *The Phantom Self* (July 12, 2013). Accessed September 23, 2015. http://phantomself.org/melanoma-journal-2/8-12-july-2013-the-second-hill/.

Dante Alighieri, "The Inferno." John Ciardi, trans. (New York: Random House, 1996).

Dawes, M., and Lens, M. B. "Global Perspectives of Contemporary Epidemiological Trends of Cutaneous Malignant Melanoma." *The British Journal of Dermatology*, 150, no.2 (2004); 179–85.

Djulbegovic, Benjamin. "Lifting the Fog of Uncertainty from the Practice of Medicine." *British Medical Journal* 329, no.7480 (December 18, 2004): 1419–20. doi : 10.1136/bmj.329.7480.1419. http://www.ncbi.nlm.nih.gov/pmc/articles/PMC535956/#ref9.

"Eligibility Criteria for Free Flights to Non-emergency Medical Appointments." *Hope Air*. Accessed September 22, 2015. http://www.hopeair.ca/FeaturePage.aspx?pgid=6&mst=~/wwd/WhatWeDo.master.

Eysenbach, Gunther. "The Impact of the Internet on Cancer Outcomes." *A Cancer Journal for Clinicians* 53, no. 6 (November/December 2003): 356–71. http://oralcancerfoundation.org/about/pdf/internet_cancer.pdf.

FDAReview.org. "The Drug Development and Approval Process." Accessed September 17, 2015. http://www.fdareview.org/approval_process.shtml .

Flanigan, Jaclyn C., Jilaveanu, Lucia B., Faries, Mark, et al. "Melanoma Brain Metastases: Is It Time to Reassess the Bias?" *Current Problems in Cancer* 35, no. 4 (July–August 2011: 200–210.

Freeman, G. J., Long, A. J., Honjo, T., et al. "Engagement of the PD-1 Immunoinhibitory Receptor by a Novel B7 Family Member Leads to Negative Regulation of Lymphocyte Activation." *The Journal of Experimental Medicine* 192, no. 7 (October 2, 2000): 1027–34. doi: 10.1084/jem.192.7.1027.

Gaffney, Alexander. "Company's Compassion Leads to Clinical Hold on Experimental Drug." *Regulatory Affairs Professional Society* (November 19, 2014). Accessed September 21, 2015. http://raps.org/Regulatory-Focus/News/2014/11/19/20780/Companys-Compassion-Leads-to-Clinical-Hold-on-Experimental-Drug/.

"Gamma Knife Surgery." *Neurological Surgery in Winnipeg*. Accessed September 23, 2015. http://www.wrha.mb.ca/prog/surgery/neurosurgery/.

Gawande, Atul. "Letting Go." *New Yorker*, August 2, 2010.

Golstein, Pierre. "A New Member of the Immunoglobulin Superfamily—CTLA-4." *Nature* 328 (July 16, 1987): 267–70. doi: 10.1038/328267a0.

Google. "Mellifluous." Accessed September 17, 2015. https://www.google.com/search?q=mellifluous&ie=utf-8&oe=utf-8.

"Health Canada Approves Yervoy (Ipilimumab) for First-line Treatment of Adults with Metastatic Melanoma, the Most Deadly Form of Skin Cancer." Bristol-Myers Squibb Canada (September 16, 2014). Accessed September 17, 2015. http://www.bmscanada.ca/en/news/releases.

Ho, Mae-Wan, and Cummins, Joe. "London Drug Trial Catastrophe—Collapse of Science and Ethics." *Institute of Science in Society* (July 4, 2006). Accessed September 23, 2015. http://www.i-sis.org.uk/LDTC.php.

Hodi, F. Stephen, O'Day, Steven J., McDermott, David F., et al. "Improved Survival with Ipilimumab in Patients with Metastatic Melanoma." *New England Journal of Medicine* 363 (August 19, 2010): 711–23. doi: 10.1056/NEJMoa1003466.

Hwang, Steven W., et al. "Adjuvant Gamma Knife Radiosurgery Following Surgical Resection of Brain Metastases: A 9-Year Retrospective Cohort Study." *Journal of Neuro-Oncology* 98, no. 1 (May 2010): 77–82.

"Immunity Let Loose." *Nature* 498 (June 13, 2013): 140–41. doi: 10.1038/498140d.

"Ipilimumab—FDA's Top 10 Blockbuster Decisions." *Fierce Biotech.* Accessed September 21, 2015. http://www.fiercebiotech.com/special-reports/fdas-top-10-blockbuster-decisions/ipilimumab-fdas-top-10-blockbuster-decisions.

"Ipilumumab." *Wikipedia.* Accessed September 23, 2015. http://en.wikipedia.org/wiki/Ipilimumab.

Ishida, Yasumasa, Agata, Yasutoshi, Honjo, Tasuku, et al. "Induced Expression of PD-1, a Novel Member of the Immunoglobulin Gene Superfamily, upon Programmed Cell Death." *EMBO Journal* (November 11, 1992): 3887–95.

Jackson, Emily. "Toronto Man Dies without Access to Bristol-Myers Squibb Experimental Drug." *The Toronto Star*, July 11, 2012.

Jäger, Elke, and Knuth, Alexander. "The Discovery of Cancer/Testis Antigens by Autologous Typing with T Cell Clones and the Evolution of Cancer Vaccines." *Cancer Immunity* 12, no. 6 (May 1, 2012).

Jagsi, Reshma, et al. "Real-Time Rationing of Scarce Resources: The Northeast Proton Therapy Center Experience." *Journal of Clinical Oncology* 22, no. 11 (June 1, 2004): 2246–50. doi : 10.1200/JCO.2004.10.083 JCO.

Jones, L. A., and Salgaller, M. L. "Immunologic Approaches to Antigen Discovery for Cancer Vaccines." Expert Opinion on Investigational Drugs 9, no. 3 (March 2000): 481–90.

Khan, Mohammad K., Khan, Niloufer, Almasan, Alex, et al. "Future of Radiation Therapy for Malignant Melanoma in an Era of Newer, More Effective Biological Agents." *Onco Targets and Therapy* 4 (August 9, 2011): 137–48. doi: 10.2147/OTT.S20257.

Latchman, Y., Wood, C. R., Chernova, T., Chaudhary, D., et al. "PD-L2 Is a Second Ligand for PD-1 and Inhibits T Cell Activation." *Nature Immunology* 3 (March 2, 2001): 261–68. PMID: 11224527.

Leach, Dana, Krummel, Matthew, and Allison, James. "Enhancement of Antitumor Immunity by CTLA-4 Blockade." *Science* 272 (March 22, 1996): 1734–36.

Lens, M. B., and Dawes, M. "Global Perspectives of Contemporary Epidemiological Trends of Cutaneous Malignant Melanoma." *The British Journal of Dermatology* 150, no. 2 (2004).

Lupkin, Sydney. "Dad Pleading for Unapproved Cancer Drug Dies." Good Morning America, November 25, 2013.

Maio M., Danielli, R., Chiarion-Sileni, V., et al. "Efficacy and Safety of Ipilimumab in Patients with Pre-treated, Uveal Melanoma." *Annals of Oncology* 24: 2911–15, no. 11 (2013). doi: 10.1093/annonc/mdt376.

Martin, Paul J. " Responsibility for Costs Associated With Clinical Trials." *Journal of Clinical Oncology* 32, no. 30 (October 20, 2014): 3357–59. doi: 10.1200/JCO.2014.57.1422 JCO. http://jco.ascopubs.org/content/32/30/3357.full.

Martinuk, Susan. *The Use of Positron Emission Tomography (PET) for Cancer Care across Canada.* Vancouver, BC: AAPS, Inc. and Triumf (2011).

McGee, Peter. *Kayak Routes of the Pacific Northwest Coast: From Northern Oregon to British Columbia's North Coast.* Vancouver: Greystone Books (2004).

McTyre, Emory, Scott, Jacob, and Chinnaiyan, Prakash. "Whole Brain Radiotherapy for Brain Metastasis." *Surgical Neurology International* 4 Suppl 4 (May 2, 2013): S236–44. doi : 10.4103/2152-7806.111301.

"Medical Services Commission Out of Province and Out of Country Medical Care Guidelines." Province of British Columbia, January 19, 2011. Accessed September 23, 2015. http://www2.gov.bc.ca/gov/DownloadAsset?assetId=5E56E19772E649E493501CCE3A40CE32&filename=ooc_funding_guidelines.pdf.

"Merck Announces Breakthrough Therapy Designation for Lambrolizumab an Investigational Antibody Therapy for Advanced Melanoma." Whitehouse Station, NJ: Merck Sharp & Dohme Corp. (April 24, 2013). Accessed September 23, 2015. http://www.mercknewsroom.com/press-release/research-and-development-news/merck-announces-breakthrough-therapy-designation-lambrol.

Mitsis, Demytra, et al. "Trends in Demographics, Incidence, and Survival in Children, Adolescents and Young Adults (AYA) with Melanoma: A Surveillance, Epidemiology and End Results (SEER) Population-based Analysis." *Journal of Clinical Oncology* 33, no.15 supplement 9058 (May 20, 2015).

"MK-3475, Background Information for the Pediatric Subcommittee of the Oncologic Drugs and Advisory Committee Meeting." November 5, 2013. http://www.fda.gov/downloads/AdvisoryCommittees/CommitteesMeetingMaterials/Drugs/OncologicDrugsAdvisoryCommittee/UCM373171.pdf.

Mulcahy, Nick. "Critical Step: Drug Slows Cognitive Loss after Radiation." Medscape Medical News (November 1, 2012). Accessed September 24, 2015. http://www.medscape.com/viewarticle/773768.

———. "Survival 81% at 1 Year with MK-3475 in Melanoma." *Medscape* (November 21, 2013). Accessed September 24, 2015. http://www.medscape.com/viewarticle/814825.

"NCCN Trends." *National Comprehensive Cancer Network* (May 2013). Accessed September 17, 2015. https://www.nccn.org/store/Products/Trends/pdf/Summary/NCCN_Trends_Metastatic_Melanoma_2013-05-01_Summary.pdf.

Ness, Sheryl M. "Cancer Survivors Struggle with Fear of Frequent Scans." Mayo Clinic, February 16, 2013. Accessed September 23, 2015. http://www.mayoclinic.org/diseases-conditions/cancer/expert-blog/cancer-and-scans/bgp-20056419.

Neuberger, Julia. "Do We Need a New Word for Patients?" *British Medical Journal* 318, no. 7200 (June 26, 1999): 1756–58.

Nguyen, Paul, et al. "Marital Status and Survival in Patients with Cancer." *American Journal of Clinical Oncology* (September 23, 2013). doi: 10.1200/JCO.2013.49.6489.

Nishimura, H., Nose, M., and Honjo, T. "Development of Lupus-like Autoimmune Diseases by Disruption of the PD-1 Gene Encoding an ITIM Motif-Carrying Immunoreceptor." *Immunity* 2 (August 11, 1999): 141–51. doi: doi.org/10.1016/S1074-7613(00)80089-8.

Oakley, Amanda, Rademaker, Marius, and Elwood, Mark. "Missed Melanomas—Comment." *The New Zealand Medical Journal* 127, no. 1398 (July 8, 2014).

O'Leary, Lizzie. "How to Negotiate Your Health Care Bills." *Marketplace* (September 13, 2013). Accessed September 23, 2015. http://www.marketplace.org/topics/your-money/health-care/how-negotiate-your-health-care-bills.

Pardoll, Drew M. "Immunology Beats Cancer: A Blueprint for Successful Translation." *Nature Immunology* 13, no. 12 (December 2012).

Patchell, Roy A., et al. "A Randomized Trial of Surgery in the Treatment of Single Metastases to the Brain." *New England Journal of Medicine* 322 (February 22, 1990): 494–500. doi : 10.1056/NEJM199002223220802.

———. " Postoperative Radiotherapy in the Treatment of Single Metastases to the Brain: A Randomized Trial. " *Journal of the American Medical Association* 280, no. 17 (November 4, 1998).

Petrella, Teresa, et al. "Canadian Perspective on the Clinical Management of Metastatic Melanoma." *New Evidence, Oncology Issue,* September 2012.

"Pfizer Announces Discontinuation of Phase III Clinical Trial for Patients with Advanced Melanoma." New York, April 1, 2008. Accessed September 23, 2015. http://press.pfizer.com/press-release/pfizer-announces-discontinuation-phase-iii-clinical-trial.

Phan, G. Q., Yang, J. C., Sherry, R. M., et al. "Cancer Regression and Autoimmunity Induced by Cytotoxic T Lymphocyte-Associated Antigen 4 Blockade in Patients with Metastatic Melanoma." *Proceedings of the National Academy of Sciences of the United States of America* 100, no. 14 (July 8, 2003): 8372–77. doi: 10.1073/pnas.1533209100.

Postow, Michael A., et al. "Immunologic Correlates of the Abscopal Effect in a Patient with Melanoma." *New England Journal of Medicine* 366 (March 8, 2012): 925–31. doi: 10.1056/NEJMoa1112824.

"President Clinton Takes New Action to Encourage Participation in Clinical Trials." (June 7, 2000). Accessed June 17, 2015. http://archive.hhs.gov/news/press/2000pres/20000607. html.

Raben, David, et al. "Stereotactic Body Radiation Therapy for Melanoma and Renal Cell Carcinoma: Impact of Single Fraction Equivalent Dose on Local Control." *Radiation Oncology* 6, no. 34 (April 2011). doi: 10.1186/1748-717X-6-34.

"Radiation Therapy Principles." The American Cancer Society. Accessed October 9, 2015. http://www.cancer.org/treatment/treatmentsandsideeffects/treatmenttypes/radiation/radiationtherapyprinciples/radiation-therapy-principles-how-does-radiation-work.

Rebecca, Vito W., Sondak, Vernon K., and Smalley, Keiran. "A Brief History of Melanoma: From Mummies to Mutations." *Melanoma Research* 22, no. 2 (April 2012): 114–22. doi: 10.1097/CMR.0b013e328351fa4d.

Ribas, Antoni, Robert, Caroline, Daud, Adil, et al. "Clinical Efficacy and Safety of Lambrolizumab (MK-3475, Anti-PD-1 Monoclonal Antibody) in Patients with Advanced Melanoma." *Journal of Clinical Oncology* 31 (2013) suppl abstr 9009. http://meetinglibrary.asco.org/content/114880-132.

Rosenthal, Elisabeth. "When Drug Trials Go Horribly Wrong." *New York Times*, April 7, 2006.

Sandburg, Carl. "Snatch of Sliphorn Jazz." *Harvest Poems*. New York: Harcourt, Brace & World, 1960.

"Search for a Cure." *Newsweek*, December 16, 1985.

Stockham, Abigail L., and Arvold, Nils D. "The Role of Radiation in the Management of Brain Metastases." *OncLive* (March 6, 2014).

"Systemic Cancer Therapy." *BC Cancer Agency* 15, no. 6 (June 2012). Accessed October 17, 2015. http://www.bccancer.bc.ca/systemic-therapy-site/Documents/UpdateJun2012_01Jun2012.pdf.

"Systemic Cancer Therapy." *BC Cancer Agency* 15, no. 10 (October 2012). Accessed October 4, 2015. http://www.bccancer.bc.ca/systemic-therapysite/Documents/UpdateOct2012_Supplement10Oct2012.pdf.

Szabo, Liz. "New Drugs Brighten Outlook for Melanoma." *USA Today*, May 29, 2013.

Taylor, Lynne. "B-MS Nivolumab to Dominate NSCLC Drug Market by 2022." *Pharma Times* (July 15, 2013). Accessed September 21, 2015. http://www.pharmatimes.com/Article/13-07-15/B-MS_nivolumab_to_dominate_NSCLC_drug_market_by_2022.aspx .

"The Fruits of Curiosity and Courage in Research." *Kyoto University Research Activities* 4, no. 4 (March 2015).

"The National Science Foundation: A Brief History." Accessed September 21, 2015. http://www.nsf.gov/about/history/nsf50/nsf8816.jsp.

Thompson, C. A., et al. "Surveillance CT Scans Are a Source of Anxiety and Fear of Recurrence in Long-term Lymphoma Survivors." *Annals of Oncology* 21, no. 11 (April 27, 2010): 2262–66. doi: 10.1093/annonc/mdq215.

Topalian, Suzanne L., Hodi, F. Stephen, Brahmer, Julie R., et al. "Safety, Activity, and Immune Correlates of Anti–PD-1 Antibody in Cancer." *New England Journal of Medicine* 366 (June 28, 2012): 2443–54. doi : 10.1056/NEJMoa1200690.

"Treatment of Metastatic Disease." Ocular Melanoma Foundation. Accessed October 2, 2015. http://www.ocularmelanoma.org/metstreatment.htm.

Vivean, Eva. "Overview of Generic Drugs and Drug Naming." *Merck Manual*. Accessed September 21, 2015. https://www.merckmanuals.com/home/drugs/brand-name-and-generic-drugs/overview-of-generic-drugs-and-drug-naming.

von Clausewitz, Carl. "On the Theory of War." In *On War*. Accessed September 23, 2015. http://www.gutenberg.org/files/1946/1946-h/1946-h.htm.

Wang, Steven. *Beating Melanoma: A Five-Step Survival Guide*. Baltimore: The Johns Hopkins University Press, 2011.

Weber, Jeffrey S., et al. "Extended Dose Ipilimumab with a Peptide Vaccine: Immune Correlates Associated with Clinical Benefit in Patients with Resected High-Risk Stage IIIc/IV Melanoma." *Clinical Cancer Research* 17, no. 4 (February 15, 2011): 896–906. doi: 10.1158/1078-0432.CCR-10-2463 .

Weintraub, Arlene. "Merck's Melanoma 'Game-Changer' Keytruda Likely to Bolster Drug Pricing Debate." *FiercePharma* (September 5, 2014). Accessed September 21, 2015. http://www.fiercepharma.com/story/mercks-melanoma-game-changer-keytruda-likely-bolster-drug-pricing-debate/2014-09-05.

Wilke, Cailin Moira, Wei, Shuang, Wang, Lin, et al. "T Cell and Antigen-Presenting Cell Subsets in the Tumor Microenvironment." In T. J. Curiel, ed., *Cancer Immunotherapy*. New York: Springer, 2013. doi: 10.1007/978-1-4614-4732-0_2.

Woolhandler S., et al. "Costs of Health Care Administration in the United States and Canada." *New England Journal of Medicine* 349 (August 21, 2003): 768–75.

Wooster, Richard, et al. "Mutations of the *BRAF* Gene in Human Cancer." *Nature* 417 (June 27, 2002): 949–54.

"World Medical Association Declaration of Helsinki—Ethical Principles for Medical Research Involving Human Subjects." 64th WMA General Assembly, Fortaleza, Brazil, October 2013.

Zhou, Yi Yvonne, Kanter, Michael H., Wang, Jian J., and Garrido, Terhilda. "Improved Quality at Kaiser Permanente through E-Mail between Physicians and Patients." *Health Affairs* 29 (July 2010): 1370–75. doi:10.1377/hlthaff.2010.0048.

INDEX

Adoptive Cell Transfer, 100
Ahmed, Rafi, ix, 153–155
Alberta Health Services, 44
Allison, James, xiii, 150, 152–153, 162, 178; CTLA-4 antibody, 71–78; discoveries about CD 28 and CTLA-4, 70–71; early influences on, 66–67; Smithville and the discovery of the T cell antigen receptor, 68–70; university and post doctorate years, 67–68
American Cancer Society, 180
American Society of Clinical Oncologists (ASCO), 143
Apoptosis. See Programmed Cell Death-1, 149
Arseneau, Flavin, 150
Auden, Nick, 170–171, 171
autoimmune disease, 71, 73, 150, 151, 156

B cell, 148
B7, 151
Barnard, Kathy, ix; advice from, 18–19, 33, 34, 37, 42, 109–110, 110, 120, 161; recovery from melanoma, 17–19, 66; support to melanoma patients, 178, 179, 180; symposium, 164
BC Cancer Agency, 12–13, 16, 19, 20, 33, 34, 37, 41, 43, 47, 54, 56, 93, 96, 99, 120, 125–126, 164, 165, 171, 179, 180, 183
BCCA. See BC Cancer Agency

Benazzo, Zaya, 3
Bernstein, Vanessa, ix, 182, 183
Beverly Hills Cancer Center, 133, 136
Blaker, Clay, 68
BRAF mutation, 18, 33, 34, 37–38, 165
brain metastases, 41, 44, 107, 108–109, 113, 122, 124, 138, 140, 188; treatments for, 109, 110, 112, 117–118, 121–126, 165–166
Breslow depth, 7
Bristol-Myers Squibb (BMS), 46, 90–91, 94; compassionate care, 18–19, 41–42, 56, 59, 170–171, 181; cost of participating in trials, 136; eligibility for trials, 91, 99, 100; recruitment, 50; Medarex and, 74; nivolumab and, 155; trial design, 42, 76
Brooks, Stan, 67

Canada Health Act, 160–161
Canadian Cancer Trials, 89
Cancer Care Alliance Center, Seattle, 90
Carnegie Institute, 148
CD28, 70–71, 72, 75, 152; super agonist, 75
Chan, Richard, 120
Chang, George, ix, 26, 30, 31–32, 34, 37, 40, 47, 51
Cheung, Winston, 164
Chinnaiyan, Prakash, 117
chronic infections, 154–155

C-KIT, 18
clinical trials, xiv, 33, 93, 153, 166, 179,
   183; access, problems with, 89, 114,
   118, 131, 133–138, 139, 181, 186;
   compassionate care, 41–42, 170–172;
   crossover option, 93–94, 94, 97, 136,
   137; ethical issues, 50–51, 170–172;
   financial assistance to patients, 136,
   160–162; open label, 93; successful,
   59, 73–77, 156, 164; uncertainty of
   result, 143–144
clinical trials, locations of: MD Anderson
   Cancer Center, 65, 68, 134; The
   Angeles Clinic, 90, 92, 94, 96, 101,
   101–104, 128, 136, 166, 167, 183;
   Beverly Hills Cancer Center, 133, 136;
   Cross Cancer Institute, Edmonton, 17,
   34, 42, 44, 45, 46, 49, 50, 93, 94, 96,
   97, 99, 100, 101, 164, 179, 185; Mayo
   Clinic, 79, 81, 134, 172; Melanoma
   Center, University of California San
   Francisco, 133; National Institutes of
   Health, 100, 148, 162, 166; Pacific
   Medical Center Research Institute, 90;
   Providence Portland Medical Center,
   90; Sloan Kettering Cancer Center, 74,
   90; START (South Texas Accelerated
   Research Therapeutics), 134, 136, 137,
   138, 142, 143, 144, 159, 166, 168, 172,
   176; University of California Los
   Angeles, 135; Yale University School of
   Medicine, 90
ClinicalTrials.gov, 89–90, 145
Clinton, Bill, 161
Cornwall, Talia, ix, 1, 6, 10, 11, 25, 28, 39,
   60, 99, 163, 165–166, 167, 187, 188
Cornwall, Tom, ix, 1, 6, 10–11, 28, 50, 54,
   55, 57, 60, 84, 99, 105, 125, 127, 140,
   141, 187, 188
Cross Cancer Institute, 17, 42, 164
CT scan, 16, 53, 57, 63, 79, 80, 127, 129,
   130, 168, 173, 179, 183
CTLA-4, 71–76, 150, 152, 156
CyberKnife, 129
Cyr, Annette, 15
CytRx, 171

dacarbazine, 56–57, 59, 102, 181, 184
Dana Farber Institute, 151

Dante, Aligieri, 100
Deacon, Nigel, ix, 181–184
DeVita Jr. Vincent, 66
dexamethasone, 110, 127
Djulbegovic, Benjamin, 45
Doherty, Darcy, 41–42

Espino, Guillermo, 135

Fawdington, Thomas, xi, xii
FDA (U.S. Food and Drug
   Administration), 76, 89–90, 155,
   171–172, 173, 184
Fred Hutchinson Cancer Research
   Center, 161
Freeman, Gordon, ix, 150–156

Gamma Knife, 109, 112, 118, 127,
   129–130, 130, 164, 165, 169, 180
Gaudette, Shannon, ix, 120–121, 126, 165
Gawande, Atul, 107–108
Gerard, Bob and Yvonne, ix, 165,
   178–180, 185, 186
Glossbrenner, Ernestine, 67, 69
Google, 7, 10, 79, 90, 109, 133
Gray, measure of radiation dose, 122, 125

Hamid, Omid, ix, 92, 96, 101, 102–105,
   108, 109, 110, 124, 133, 134, 135–138,
   183
Hayaishi, Osamu, 148
Health Canada, 18–19, 20, 37, 45–46, 56,
   88, 89, 171
Health Sciences Centre, Winnipeg,
   109–110, 180
Hodi, Stephen, 76
Honjo, Tasuku, ix, xiii, 147–150, 151, 156,
   178
Human Genome Project, 151
hyperbaric oxygen therapy, 119

IL-2. See interleukin-2
immunotherapies, xiii, xiv, 17–18, 45, 56,
   61, 65, 66, 67, 73, 74–75, 77, 77–78,
   89, 93, 94, 109, 113, 114, 129, 132,
   133, 135, 146, 155, 156, 164–165, 166,
   168, 169, 173, 181, 183, 185. See also
   ipilimumab, nivolumab,
   pembrolizumab, lambrolizumab,

interferon, interleukin-2
interferon, xii, 16, 17–18, 20, 32, 38, 152
interleukin-2, 17–18, 65
ipilimumab (ipi): approval of, 19, 172;
    clinical trials of, 34, 41–42, 44, 45–46,
    56–57, 73–78, 95, 137; discovery of,
    65, 71–73; efficacy, 89, 156, 165, 173;
    treatment with, 18, 20, 37, 58–60, 60,
    63, 80, 81, 88, 93, 102, 159, 171
Ishida, Yasumasa, 148

Jagsi, Reshma, 51
Jiminez, Isabel, 134, 135, 137
Johns Hopkins, 155

Keytruda,, 173. *See also* lambrolizumab,
    pembrolizumab, MK-3475
Kim-Sing, Charmaine, ix, 43–44, 44,
    46–47, 51, 58, 87–88, 89, 112, 117,
    120–121, 125–126, 128, 131
Klimo, Paul, 17, 163
Krummel, Max, 71

lambrolizumab (lambro): clinical trials,
    89–91, 92, 93, 94, 95, 101, 102,
    133–134, 136, 137, 138, 145, 162;
    efficacy, 89, 102, 143, 164, 167;
    approval, 89, 173. *See also*
    pembrolizumab, Keytruda, MK3475
Leach, Dana, 71
Lions Gate Hospital, 30, 34, 47, 55, 59,
    60, 79, 92, 110, 112, 113, 138
Loiselle, Chris, 123, 124

Mak, Tak, 149
Martin, Paul, 161–162
MD Anderson Cancer Center, 65, 68, 134
Medarex, 73, 74, 75, 153, 155
Medical Services Plan of BC, 136, 160
Mehta, Vivek, ix, 119, 121–124, 125, 128
MEK, 165
Melanoma: adjuvant therapy, 37–38, 45,
    59, 95; etymology, xi; incidence, xiv,
    50, 164; nodular, 7, 8, 165, 179, 184;
    ocular, 181, 181–184; staging, 14, 15,
    30, 41, 51, 73, 76, 80; survival from, xii,
    7–8, 14, 19, 43–44, 46, 75–76, 171,
    181, 183
memantine, 119, 123

Merck, 91, 167; compassionate care, 170;
    consent form, 102; costs of
    participating in trials, 136, 161;
    products, 89, 90, 156, 170, 173;
    National Service Center, 133–134;
    protocols, 137, 138, 144, 145, 168, 173
MK-3475, : approval, 172, 173

clinical trials, 102, 135, 143, 144, 159, 170,
    171–172; efficacy, 165, 166, 167, 168,
    169; side effects, 143–144, 163,
    172–173, 173. *See also* pembrolizu-
    mab, lambrolizumab, Keytruda

Monopoli, Sara, 107
MRI, 16, 96, 102, 103–104, 109–111, 120,
    121, 123, 124, 126, 127–129, 131, 134,
    136, 138–139, 140, 164, 167, 169

Nakano, Toro, 149
National Academy of Sciences, 73
National Comprehensive Cancer
    Network, 184
National Science Foundation, 150
NCT01295827, 90–91, 92, 93, 135
needle biopsy, 22, 47
Nelson, Willie, 68
Neuberger, Julia, 185–186
Nishimura, Hiroshi, 149–150
nivolumab, 90; clinical trials, 93, 97, 100,
    133, 135, 155; compassionate care,
    41–42; efficacy, 155
North Shore Imaging, 138, 139, 140

Ono Pharmaceuticals, 155
Opdivo. *See* nivolumab
Osaka University, 148

Patchell, Roy 117
Patient Protection and Affordable Care
    Act, 162
patient support groups for melanoma:
    Melanoma Network of Canada, 15;
    Melanoma Research Foundation, 42,
    184; Save Your Skin Foundation, 17,
    164, 178, 180–181, 184
PD-1, 89, 110, 148–150, 151–153,
    154–155; anti-PD-1, 89, 90, 105, 109,
    110, 114, 122, 124, 131, 134, 156, 170,

171
PD-1 blockade. *See* anti PD-1
PDL-1, 151–153
PDL-2, 151
Pembrolizumab: approval of, 173. *See also* Keytruda, lambrolizumab, MK3475
PET scan, 23, 26, 30, 32, 37, 47–48, 48, 53, 80, 81, 84, 87, 92, 96, 99, 121, 128–129, 166, 173
Petrella, Teresa, 50, 161
Pfizer, 75
Phantom Self, 3, 47, 52, 57–58, 62–63, 101, 131–132, 140, 143–144, 187–188
Programmed Cell Death-1. *See* PD-1

radiation, xii, xiv; axillary area, 37, 43–44, 46, 47, 51, 53, 54, 55, 57, 58, 61, 62; brain metastases, and, 104, 105, 109, 112, 113; clinical trials with, 44–45; radiosensitizers, and, 119, 123; stereotactic, 109, 118, 122, 123, 124–125, 126, 128, 129, 164, 179–180; synergy with other treatments, 44, 77; whole brain (WBRT), 100, 117–119, 120, 122–123, 125, 125–126, 128, 145, 165, 179
Rasco, Drew, 168
Ribas, Tony, 173
Rosenberg, Steven, 65

Sahjpaul, Ramesh, ix, 112, 112–113, 113, 113–114, 128
Sandburg, Carl, 166
Sato, Takimi, 182–183
Scott, Robert, ix, 4, 9–10, 13, 16, 35, 36, 47, 48, 51, 81, 167, 184
seroma, 40, 46, 58, 61, 126
Sheridan Lake, 39, 57–59, 61, 84, 162–163, 188
Shibatani, Atsuhiro, 148
Smiljanic, Sasha, ix, xiv, xv, 16, 34, 35, 36, 41, 43, 53, 163, 181; first appointment with, 36–37; radiation, views on, 43–44; systemic therapy, efforts to obtain, 45–46, 56, 88, 92–94, 94, 96, 97, 101, 104, 105, 122, 124, 138–139, 145; metastasis, response to, 79–81, 81, 82, 92, 99, 108–109, 110, 112, 132

Smylie, Michael, 17–18, 42, 93, 97, 164–165, 179
Steinbeck, John, 62
SUV, standard uptake values, 128–129
Swedish Medical Center, 48, 49, 99, 121, 124, 129, 130

T cells, 100, 143, 143–144; antigen receptors, 69–73, 77, 156; benefits and risks, 168, 172–173; CTLA-4 "brake", 71–73; exhaustion, 154–155; memory, 78, 154; PD-1 "brake" on, 89, 148, 149–150; PD-1 regulators, 151–153, 166, 178; selection of, 148
thyroid stimulating hormone, 172
Tolcher, Tony, ix, 159, 161, 164, 166, 168, 172–173, 176; early influences, 142–144; ethical issues and solutions, views on, 170, 171–172
Topalian, Suzanne, 155
Truman, Harry, 150
Turnham, Tim, 162, 184

ultrasound, 40, 47, 80
University of British Columbia (UBC), 3, 10, 27, 50, 181
University of California Berkeley, 70, 71
University of Kyoto, 147, 148
University of Texas at Austin, 67–68, 150

Vermeulin, Sandra, ix, 128–130
von Clausewitz, Carl, 45

Wang, Steven, 32, 51, 63
Wilson, Laura, 138
Wolchuk, Jedd, 76

X-ray, 15, 16, 54, 55, 95, 102

Yervoy,. *See* ipilimumab 18

Zelboraf, 18, 37, 44
Zhou, Youwen, ix; first appointment, 13–16, 19; spread of melanoma, response to, 21, 22, 23, 26, 30, 31, 32–33, 35

ABOUT THE AUTHOR

Claudia Cornwall, a freelance writer for over twenty-five years, has written six books and many magazine articles. Her memoir, *Letter from Vienna: A Daughter Uncovers Her Family's Jewish Past*, won a BC Book prize for best nonfiction. Her biography, *At the World's Edge: Curt Lang's Vancouver, 1937–1998*, was a finalist for the 2012 Vancouver Book Award. Her medical history, *Catching Cancer: The Quest for Its Viral and Bacterial Causes*, was selected by the American Library Association's *Booklist* as one of the best books of 2013 and was short-listed for the Canadian Science Writers' Association Book Awards (2013). Claudia also teaches in Simon Fraser University's Writer's Studio.